GALVESTON DIET COOKBOOK FOR BEGINNERS

Explore a Rich Collection of Hormone Balancing and Anti-Inflammatory Recipes; Crafted for Menopausal Health, with a 60-Day Meal Plan to Guide Your Journey

Elodie Vance

TABLE OF CONTENTS

1.Embarking on a New Journey

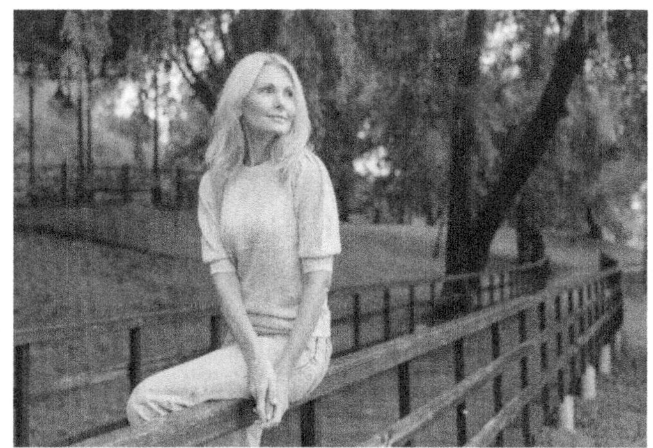

Welcome to the beginning of a transformative journey that transcends the ordinary scope of diet books. Aimed specifically at navigating the turbulent waters of menopause, this chapter is more than a starting point—it is a comprehensive embrace of change, designed uniquely for you.

As we embark on this path together, understanding the profound shifts that menopause brings to your life—both physiological and emotional—is crucial. It's essential to acknowledge how these changes impact your metabolism and overall well-being. Menopause isn't merely a phase marked by an end to menstruation but a new era where your body demands a renewed focus on balance and care.

Here, you will learn not just about the metabolic implications of menopause but how to harmonize your hormones through tailored nutritional strategies. These aren't generic eating suggestions; these are scientifically backed strategies designed to soothe inflammation, a common yet often overlooked culprit that exacerbates menopausal symptoms.

We'll also delve into psychological preparation because approaching dietary changes with the right mindset is pivotal. Think of this as setting the stage for success; it's about creating a supportive mental framework that empowers you to embrace and sustain the dietary adjustments you will learn about in the following pages.

This isn't merely a diet—it's a rekindling of vitality and health, promising to guide you with practical, family-friendly meals that cater not just to your needs but to the culinary enjoyment of your entire household. Each recipe and guide in this book respects the complex interaction between body, mind, and emotions during menopause, transforming everyday eating into a joyful, health-focused ritual.

Let's move forward, not just with the hope of managing symptoms, but with the goal of thriving through menopause, wielding our diet as a powerful tool for holistic well-being. Every bite, every ingredient in this journey is chosen to bring harmony to your body in its profound time of change. Are you ready to take this step into a healthful future? The journey begins now.

Decoding Menopause and Its Metabolic Impact

Menopause marks a significant phase in a woman's life; it's not just an end to fertility, but a beginning to a profound shift in her body's internal workings, particularly her metabolic health. To understand and navigate these changes adeptly, it's essential to first decode what menopause entails and how it impacts metabolism, a core aspect of our holistic well-being.

Menopause naturally occurs as a part of aging and is diagnosed after 12 consecutive months without a menstrual period. The age at which it happens varies, typically between 45 and 55 years, but the changes that come with it are almost universal. Hormones like estrogen and progesterone, vital players in a woman's reproductive years, begin to decline. This hormonal adjustment doesn't just pause the menstrual cycle; it shifts the entire metabolic rate of the body, influencing everything from how quickly calories are burned to how fats are stored.

Estrogen, particularly, has been like a conductor in the orchestra of the female body, influencing mood, weight, and energy. As its levels drop, you might find it harder to manage weight despite sticking to diets that worked before. This bewildering fluctuation is because your body now responds differently to fats, carbohydrates, and proteins. Typically, there's an increase in abdominal fat—a type notorious for its role in promoting inflammatory processes and various chronic diseases.

This metabolic slowdown isn't just about aesthetics or discomfort. It heightens the risk for several conditions like type 2 diabetes, heart disease, and osteoporosis, making menopausal dietary management not just about maintaining weight but about enhancing long-term health and vitality.

Understanding these changes, one wonders: How can we counteract this slowing metabolism? The solution lies in an anti-inflammatory diet rich in nutrients that can help stabilize these hormonal fluctuations and promote metabolic health. By focusing on hormone-balancing foods and avoiding triggers that can cause inflammation, you can significantly mitigate these effects.

Let's consider insulin sensitivity, which often decreases during menopause. A diet high in refined sugars and carbohydrates can exacerbate insulin resistance and lead to weight gain and other health issues. Instead, emphasizing a balanced intake of complex carbohydrates, high-quality proteins, and healthy fats can support stable blood sugar levels and a steady metabolic rate.

Vegetables, fruits, whole grains, and lean proteins contain the essential vitamins, minerals, and antioxidants that combat inflammation. Foods rich in omega-3 fatty acids, like salmon and flaxseeds, are particularly beneficial. They not only help in reducing inflammation but also support brain health, which can be crucial during menopause, a time when many women experience foggy thinking and memory lapses.

Equally important is hydration. Water plays a critical role in maintaining metabolic functions and aiding digestion and nutrient absorption. It becomes even more crucial during menopause, as changes in the body can lead to dryness and the sensation of overheating. Keeping hydrated helps regulate body temperature and supports overall cellular health.

Furthermore, engaging in regular physical activity can complement dietary efforts to boost metabolism. Exercise helps build muscle mass, which naturally declines with age. Since muscle burns more calories than fat, increasing muscle mass through activities like resistance training can counteract the metabolic slowdown.

Apart from diet and exercise, stress management also has a significant role in managing metabolic health during menopause. Stress can lead to overeating and choosing less nutritious foods, which can aggravate metabolic and hormonal imbalances. Techniques such as mindfulness, yoga, or even simple breathing exercises can be effective in maintaining hormonal equilibrium and enhancing emotional well-being.

Lastly, sleep cannot be overlooked. Quality sleep is crucial, especially now, as it helps regulate the hormones that affect appetite and stress. Establishing a soothing bedtime routine, reducing screen time before bed, and creating a restful environment can foster better sleep, thus supporting metabolic and overall health.

In summary, while menopause can be a challenging time due to various physical and emotional changes, understanding its impact on metabolism and adopting a tailored, nourishing diet can transform this phase into one of renewal and positive health. By focusing on anti-inflammatory, nutrient-dense foods, staying hydrated, maintaining an active lifestyle, managing stress, and prioritizing good sleep, you can support your body's metabolic health and continue to thrive through menopause and beyond.

This holistic approach doesn't just address the symptoms but enriches your quality of life, proving that menopause can indeed be a powerful impetus for embracing a healthier, more balanced lifestyle. Through informed choices and mindful eating, you can transform this natural progression into a rejuvenating journey toward sustained well-being. This is not merely about making it through menopause but flourishing during it and after. Embrace this opportunity to nourish and care for your body as it adapts and transforms, and you'll uncover a path that is as rewarding as it is healthy.

Key Strategies for Hormonal Equilibrium

Achieving hormonal equilibrium during menopause can feel like trying to balance on a moving seesaw. Just as you think you've found stability, a shift occurs, tossing your well-being into the air. However, with the right strategies, you can regain control and possibly even enjoy the ride. This section delves into practical, actionable tips that not only aim to balance your hormones but also enhance your overall vitality during menopause.

Hormonal equilibrium in menopause isn't about restoring your body to its pre-menopausal state; rather, it's about creating a new internal environment where health can flourish despite hormonal fluctuations. Given the complexity of hormonal interaction, a multifaceted approach is necessary, focusing on diet, lifestyle, and mental well-being.

1. Nutrition: Fuel for Hormonal Health

First, let's discuss dietary adjustments. Carbohydrates, protein, and fat all have roles in hormone regulation. A diet low in processed foods and high in phytoestrogens, fiber, and omega-3 fatty acids can support hormonal balance. Phytoestrogens, found in flaxseeds, soy products, and sesame seeds, mimic the effects of estrogen and can help stabilize estrogen levels. Fiber aids in digestion and excretion, helping clear excess hormones from the body, while omega-3 fatty acids reduce inflammation, which can exacerbate hormonal disturbances.

2. Active Lifestyle: More Than Just Weight Management

Physical activity is another cornerstone of achieving hormonal equilibrium. Regular exercise, particularly strength training and aerobic workouts, can mitigate insulin resistance, improve mood, reduce stress, and help maintain muscle mass, which naturally declines with age. Exercise also stimulates the production of endorphins, the body's natural painkillers and mood elevators, thus providing a natural antidote to the emotional rollercoasters often experienced during menopause.

3. Sleep: Underrated Yet Vital

Sleep and hormonal balance are deeply interconnected. Lack of sleep can disrupt the secretion of cortisol, often referred to as the stress hormone, which in turn affects other hormones, including insulin. Establishing a calming bedtime routine, prioritizing a cool, dark, and quiet sleep environment, and possibly incorporating practices such as meditation or gentle yoga can significantly improve sleep quality.

4. Stress Reduction: Calming the Hormonal Storm

Stress management is critical in maintaining hormonal equilibrium. Chronic stress can lead to elevated cortisol levels, disrupting the delicate balance of hormones. Techniques such as deep breathing, mindfulness meditation, and regular physical activity can effectively reduce stress. Furthermore, engaging in hobbies and maintaining social connections can also provide emotional support and stress relief.

5. Supplementation: When Diet Isn't Enough

While getting most nutrients from food is ideal, certain supplements may be beneficial in supporting hormonal health during menopause. For instance, vitamin D, often lacking in the diet, is crucial for bone health, especially as the decline in estrogen during menopause increases the risk for osteoporosis. Similarly, magnesium supplements can improve sleep and reduce hot flashes.

6. Herbal Support: A Natural Approach

Several herbs have been noted for their potential to support hormonal balance. Black cohosh, for example, has been widely studied for its ability to reduce menopausal symptoms such as hot flashes and mood disturbances. However, it's essential to consult with a healthcare provider before starting any herbal regimen, as herbs can interact with medications and aren't suitable for everyone.

7. Mindfulness and Emotional Well-being

Emotional health is perhaps one of the most overlooked aspects of hormonal balance. Hormones can directly impact your mood, and your mood can, in turn, influence hormone levels, creating a cycle that can be difficult to break. Practices such as journaling, mindfulness, and therapy can be valuable tools for emotional regulation. Acknowledging and addressing emotional needs can help maintain hormonal balance by reducing stress and enhancing your overall quality of life.

8. Engaging with Professional Guidance

Finally, while self-care is incredibly important, engaging with professionals who specialize in menopausal health can provide personalized insights into managing hormonal changes. Endocrinologists, nutritionists, and menopausal specialists can offer guidance based on your specific health needs and conditions.

In essence, achieving hormonal equilibrium during menopause is about more than just managing symptoms—it's about embracing a holistic approach to health that incorporates thoughtful nutrition, regular physical activity, sufficient sleep, stress management, possible supplementation, herbal aids, emotional well-being, and professional guidance. This comprehensive approach ensures that you not only address the hormonal changes occurring in your body but also enhance your overall health and well-being, turning menopause from a challenge into an opportunity for growth and renewal.

Nutritional Strategies for Menopausal Well-being

Navigating through the menopausal transition, you might find that foods which once felt fulfilling no longer serve you the same way. Our bodies in menopause require a refined strategy that hinges greatly on nutritional adjustments to cater to the evolving needs of slowing metabolism and hormonal oscillations. This sub-chapter delves into the specifics of constructing a nutritional plan that doesn't just aim to soothe symptoms but enhances overall well-being throughout menopause and beyond.

Understanding the Menopausal Shift in Nutrient Needs

As estrogen levels plummet, the risk of cardiovascular disease and osteoporosis rises, steering the focus towards nutrients that support heart and bone health. Calcium, vitamin D, magnesium, and vitamin K2 become crucial. Each plays a distinctive role, from bolstering bone density to enhancing heart function. Furthermore, as metabolism slows, adjusting caloric intake becomes necessary to avoid unwanted weight gain, yet this must be balanced carefully to maintain muscle mass and vigor.

Fats – Choosing the Right Type

Contrary to popular belief, not all fats are foes. During menopause, healthy fats found in avocados, nuts, seeds, and oily fish become particularly beneficial. These fats are not only pivotal for hormonal health, providing the necessary components from which our bodies can craft hormones, but are also fundamental in combating inflammation—an often silent accomplice in menopausal discomforts.

Protein – Vital for Muscle Maintenance

Maintaining muscle mass is crucial as it naturally dwindles with age and hormonal changes. Ensuring adequate protein intake supports muscle repair and synthesis. It also aids in feeling fuller for longer, which can help manage weight by curbing the mid-meal hunger pangs that lead to overeating. Incorporate diverse protein sources, from lean meats to plant-based options like lentils and quinoa, to keep meals both interesting and nourishing.

Carbohydrates – Selecting Wisely

It's not about eliminating carbohydrates but choosing them wisely. During menopause, it's advisable to reduce high-glycemic carbs which spike blood sugar levels and can exacerbate hormonal fluctuations. Instead, focus on fiber-rich vegetables and whole grains. These not only help maintain a healthy digestive system but their slow-releasing energy helps in managing insulin sensitivity, a common concern during menopause.

Hydration – Often Overlooked but Crucial

Water consumption might seem like elementary advice, yet it remains one of the most overlooked aspects of a menopausal diet. Adequate hydration aids in regulating body temperature—a boon considering the hot flashes and night sweats. It also supports kidney function and can help reduce bloating, which some women experience due to hormonal changes.

Addressing Common Menopausal Symptoms with Nutrition

Hot Flashes and Heart Health

Foods rich in phytoestrogens, such as flaxseeds and soy, can mimic the effects of estrogen in the body and may help balance hormones naturally. Regarding heart health, incorporating antioxidants and potassium-rich foods like berries and bananas can support blood pressure regulation and cardiovascular well-being.

Bone Health

With the risk of osteoporosis heightened during and after menopause, calcium-rich foods such as dairy, greens like kale and broccoli, and fortified plant milk should be a staple in your diet. However, calcium's role isn't standalone as vitamin D is critical for calcium absorption. Thus, ensuring enough sunlight exposure or considering a vitamin D supplement becomes crucial.

The Emotional Connection to Eating

Menopause can also be a time of significant emotional upheaval, and how we eat can reflect our emotional states. Emotional eating can be mitigated by maintaining a diet that stabilizes blood sugar levels, thus avoiding the dramatic spikes and dips that can affect your mood. Incorporating foods rich in omega-3 fatty acids, like fish and walnuts, can support brain health and potentially alleviate mood swings.

Building a Menopause-Friendly Kitchen

Creating an environment that supports these dietary goals starts with how we stock our kitchen. Replace easily accessible junk food with healthy snacks like almonds and carrots. Plan meals ahead to avoid last-minute decisions that might not align with nutritional goals. Keep it varied to cover all nutrient bases and to keep the diet interesting and enjoyable, which is crucial for long-term adherence.

Embracing this comprehensive nutritional strategy during menopause is not merely about adapting to bodily changes but about welcoming a phase of life with vitality and enthusiasm. By understanding how our bodies' needs evolve during this time, and adjusting our dietary habits accordingly, we can alleviate many of the physical discomforts of menopause and emerge healthily, feeling balanced and rejuvenated.

Beginning Steps: Psychologically Preparing for Dietary Success

Embarking on a dietary journey, particularly during menopause, is no small feat. It's a voyage that demands not only physical adjustment but profound psychological readiness. We often underestimate the power of our mental state in determining the success of any dietary change. Hence, gearing up psychologically is a crucial beginning step for ensuring dietary success throughout menopause.

Understanding the Impact of Change

Menopause is a period marked by significant changes, not just physically but in every aspect of life. Adjusting your diet during this time can feel daunting. Acknowledging the challenges and accepting that difficulties are part of the journey can equip you with a resilient mindset. It's beneficial to understand that dietary changes aren't about stringent restrictions or quick fixes but sustainable habits that nurture your body.

Setting Realistic Expectations

One common pitfall in any diet adjustment is setting goals that are either too vague or unrealistically high. "I will eat healthier" is a noble starting point, but it lacks specificity and measurability. Instead, articulate what exactly "eating healthier" looks like in actionable terms—perhaps it's incorporating a serving of vegetables in every meal, or reducing processed sugar intake by half. Setting realistic and precise goals can lead to a more focused and manageable plan, providing clear milestones and a sense of achievement.

Cultivating a Positive Relationship with Food

Menopause can often distort our body image and how we interact with food. Viewing food as either a friend or foe can lead to a fraught relationship where eating becomes a source of stress. It's important to cultivate a perspective of food as nourishment, a source of vitality, and a way to celebrate our bodies. Emphasizing this positive interaction involves appreciating the flavors, enjoying the process of meal preparation, and acknowledging the nourishment each meal provides.

Building a Support System

Just as you would pack essentials for a long trip, preparing for a dietary shift means assembling a support system. This network could include friends who uplift you, family members who understand your goals, or online communities of women who are on a similar path. Sharing your struggles, successes, and insights can make the journey less intimidating and more of a shared experience.

Mindfulness and Emotional Eating

Mindfulness—an awareness of the present moment, characterized by acceptance—can be an extremely effective tool in managing how you eat. It involves paying attention to hunger and fullness cues, eating without distraction, and recognizing emotional eating triggers. During menopause, emotional fluctuations are common and can often lead to eating in response to feelings rather than hunger. Mindfulness helps distinguish between the two, enabling more thoughtful food choices.

Anticipating and Managing Setbacks

Setbacks are an inevitable part of any change process, including dietary adjustments. Anticipating that there will be moments of weakness or deviation allows you to develop strategies to navigate these effectively. Rather than viewing them as failures, treat setbacks as learning opportunities. Analyzing what led to the slip and strategizing ways to handle similar situations in the future can strengthen your dietary practice.

Flexibility Over Rigidity

No matter how well you plan, the unpredictable nature of life means things will not always go according to that plan. Flexibility—both in mindset and action—is key. If a particular dietary change isn't working, be it due to taste preferences, physical reactions, or lifestyle constraints, it's alright to reevaluate and adjust your course.

Visualizing Success

Visualization is a powerful technique where you imagine completing a task successfully. Picturing yourself thriving on your new diet, imagining how you'll feel, and what you'll be doing can inspire and motivate. Visualization solidifies the belief in your ability to succeed and brings your goals within reach, making the dietary transition an integral part of your life rather than a distant or disconnected chore.

Gradual Changes Rather Than Overhauls

The allure of instant transformation is strong, but sudden and comprehensive changes are usually unsustainable in the long term. Incorporating gradual adjustments—adding a new healthy habit every week or substituting one meal a day with a healthier option—can lead to more enduring changes, reducing the feeling of overwhelm and giving the body and mind time to adapt.

Acknowledging the Journey Ahead

Finally, embracing this dietary shift is acknowledging a journey. It's about setting out with a map—the plan you've crafted—knowing the destination but being open to the paths that lead there. Each step, each choice is a part of adapting to a new way of life that prioritizes your well-being through menopause and beyond.

In preparing psychologically for dietary success during menopause, you are doing much more than altering what you eat. You're fundamentally redefining your lifestyle to harmonize with your body's needs in a period of significant change. This transformation, grounded in both mental and physical readiness, is not just about enduring menopause but thriving through it with health, joy, and confidence.

2.Delving into Intermittent Fasting

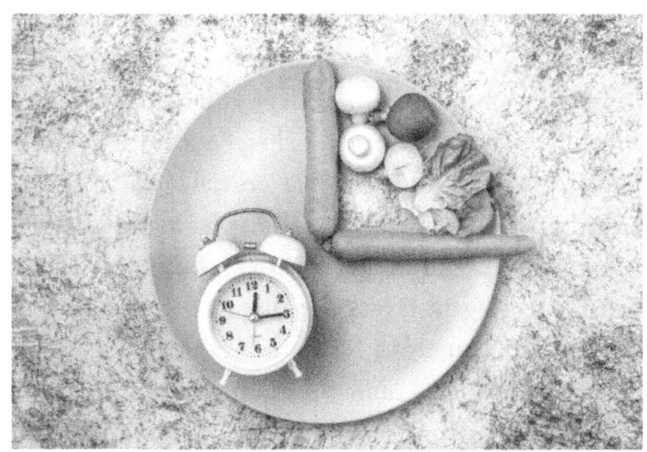

As we journey through the explorative path of menopausal health, one strategy that emerges with compelling benefits is intermittent fasting. Unlike many trends that flicker brightly but briefly in the wellness landscape, intermittent fasting—or time-restricted feeding—owns a storied history rooted in both ancient practices and modern science. But what makes it particularly appealing for women in menopause?

When we talk about metabolism during menopause, many of you have shared stories of how your once predictable bodily responses now seem to play a bewildering game of hide and seek. It's here that intermittent fasting steps in—not as a strict instructor, but as a guide, helping to reestablish a rhythm in an otherwise erratic metabolic dance.

Imagine this: your body, accustomed to the continuous task of processing food, suddenly finds a period of rest, a brief but profound silence in the symphony of digestion. This pause—a fundamental aspect of intermittent fasting—allows cells to repair, focus on detoxifying, and improve their sensitivity to insulin, pivotal during the insulin-resistant phase of menopause.

The beauty of this approach lies not just in its simplicity, but also in its adaptability. Many express concerns around the rigidity of diet regimes, fearing a loss of social joy and culinary delight. Yet, intermittent fasting promises flexibility. It's less about eliminating your favorite dishes and more about reshaping the clock—when you eat becomes as significant as what you eat. This method can effortlessly blend into your life, encouraging a mindful relationship with food, without the strain of drastic dietary overhauls.

Moreover, delving into this practice isn't merely a solo journey. It's about creating space in your schedule where your body can embrace healing naturally, allowing you to enjoy those cherished moments of meals with family and friends more knowingly and healthfully.

So, as we prepare to weave intermittent fasting into your daily routine, consider it not just a dietary adjustment, but a stepping stone to reclaiming control over your bodily rhythms and wellbeing—a truly empowering tool in your menopausal health toolkit.

Advantages of Time-Restricted Feeding

Embracing time-restricted feeding, a core component of intermittent fasting, offers an intriguing array of benefits, especially for women navigating the complex shifts of menopause. This approach, centered around timing rather than caloric restriction, aligns beautifully with our bodies' intrinsic rhythms—providing a gentle nudge to metabolism, enhancing overall health, and contributing to hormonal equilibrium. Here, we delve into a detailed exploration of how this practice can become a transformative part of your health regimen.

Metabolic Revival

The onset of menopause often brings about a significant impact on metabolism. You might find that the diets which worked in your thirties or forties suddenly seem ineffective. Time-restricted feeding steps into this scenario as a metabolic reviver. By confining eating to a specific window—commonly 8-10 hours a day—you encourage your body to enter a state of fasting for the remaining 14-16 hours. This shift from constant energy intake compels the body to tap into stored fat for energy, a process termed as lipolysis, which is crucial for weight management during menopause.

During these fasting periods, the lowered levels of insulin also facilitate cellular repair processes, effectively giving your body the cue to focus on maintenance instead of growth. This response is vital for longevity and health, particularly when hormonal changes can predispose one to age-related diseases.

Enhanced Hormonal Harmony

Hormonal fluctuations are the linchpins in the menopausal experience, often leading to symptoms like hot flashes, night sweats, and mood swings. Time-restricted feeding can symbiotically enhance your body's natural hormone regulation. By improving insulin sensitivity during fasting periods, this eating pattern helps stabilize blood sugar levels, indirectly aiding in the management of estrogen levels. Stable blood sugar and insulin levels mean less stress on the body, allowing other hormones to more easily find their balance.

Moreover, fasting increases levels of human growth hormone (HGH), which helps in maintaining muscle mass—a common concern as you age. Muscle is metabolically active, which not only helps in maintaining a healthy weight but also supports hormone synthesis and degradation.

Improvements in Sleep Quality

Many menopausal women find that sleep evades them just when they need it the most. This can be a byproduct of weight gain, hormonal imbalances, or increased stress levels. Interestingly, aligning your eating schedule with your circadian rhythm through time-restricted feeding can lead to significant improvements in sleep quality. Eating earlier in the day aligns food intake with your natural cortisol rhythms, ensuring that energy levels wind down naturally towards the evening, promoting restful sleep.

As sleep quality improves, so does the regulation of hormones like cortisol and melatonin, which further aids in managing menopausal symptoms effectively. Better sleep also means better mood and cognitive function, so the benefits are comprehensive and deeply impactful.

Cardiovascular Health

Postmenopausal women often face an increased risk of developing cardiovascular diseases. Time-restricted feeding enhances heart health by influencing various biomarkers such as blood pressure, cholesterol levels, and inflammatory markers. Fasting periods help reduce LDL (bad) cholesterol and triglycerides, crucial elements that contribute to the thickening or hardening of arteries. Moreover, the anti-inflammatory effects of fasting can protect against vascular diseases. Inflammation can lead to numerous health issues, including heart diseases, and by limiting eating to a specific timeframe, you're essentially giving your body a better chance to fight inflammation more effectively.

Cognitive Clarity and Emotional Well-being

The impact of dietary practices on mental health cannot be understated, especially during menopause, when many women report feeling less sharp or more forgetful. Fasting has been shown to increase brain-derived neurotrophic factor (BDNF), a protein that plays a critical role in learning, memory, and the generation of new neurons. By boosting brain health, you not only tackle the immediate concerns around menopause-induced fog but also park a solid defense against longer-term cognitive decline.

Emotionally, aligning your eating patterns with biological rhythms can enhance your sense of control and well-being. Many women report a significant boost in mood and reduced anxiety when their bodies adapt to a time-restricted feeding regimen. The discipline of fasting, surprisingly, can lead to a liberating feeling, reducing the paradoxical stress around eating and food choices by simplifying decisions.

Practical Integration

Now, the practical side might initially seem intimidating. How do you adjust to a confined eating window without feeling restricted or socially isolated? The key lies in gradual adaptation. Start by limiting late-night snacking, slowly bringing your dinner times forward. Align social engagements around brunch or lunch rather than late dinners. Make your first meal wholesome and satisfying, so you are energized for the day without overwhelming cravings.

Integration into your lifestyle needs to be seamless—more a gentle shift than an abrupt change. Observing how your body and mind respond as you tweak your eating windows will provide invaluable insights into what your optimal pattern might be.

In conclusion, time-restricted feeding isn't just about when you eat; it's a profound step towards syncing your dietary rhythm with your body's natural needs, particularly during the transitional phase of menopause. By focusing on the timing of meals, you can unlock a series of beneficial metabolic, hormonal, and psychological changes, fostering not just immediate well-being but also long-term health. So, embrace this practice with openness and curiosity, and watch as it transforms not just your diet, but your overall approach to health during menopause.

Guidelines for Initiating Intermittent Fasting

Embarking on the intermittent fasting journey is an adventure in redefining not only the way we eat but also how we view our relationship with food—particularly pertinent during the menopause transition. It requires an understanding that initiating and sustaining fasting isn't merely a diet but a lifestyle change that promises significant benefits. Here's a comprehensive guide to starting intermittent fasting, illuminated by careful research and practical experience.

Understanding Your Baseline

Before diving into intermittent fasting, it's crucial to assess your current dietary habits. Reflect on your typical eating times, the nature of your meals, and how your body feels daily. Are your meals spread out, or do you tend to eat in a defined window already? Understanding this baseline will not only help in setting realistic expectations but also in customizing your fasting plan to suit your unique needs.

Choosing Your Fasting Window

One of the first steps is determining the fasting method that resonates with your lifestyle and physical needs. A popular approach is the 16/8 method, where you eat during an 8-hour window and fast for 16 hours. However, for beginners, especially during menopause when the body is already undergoing several adjustments, you might consider starting with a gentler regimen like 12/12 and gradually working your way up as your body adapts.

Gradual Introduction

Introducing intermittent fasting gradually can help mitigate some initial discomfort such as hunger pangs or slight headaches, common as the body shifts from glucose to fat for energy. Begin by delaying breakfast an hour later than usual and having dinner an hour earlier. This incremental adjustment helps your body smoothly transition into a state of fasting without severe stress or shock.

Mindful Eating

During your eating window, focus on nutrient-dense foods that support menopausal health. Prioritize vegetables, lean proteins, and healthy fats that not only fulfill your nutritional needs but also keep you satiated longer, easing the fasting periods. This focus helps combat common nutrient deficiencies that can arise during menopause and ensures that your body is fortified with the necessary resources to function optimally.

Hydration Focus

Hydration is a cornerstone of any dietary change, particularly important in fasting. Water aids in appetite control and helps reduce some common side effects of fasting like headaches and fatigue. Aim to drink plenty of water throughout your eating window and try to include hydrating foods in your meals. Herbal teas, which are calorie-free, can be a comforting and hydrating choice during fasting hours.

Listen to Your Body

Initiating intermittent fasting during menopause should be approached with a heightened sense of awareness towards one's body. Pay attention to how you feel during different times of the day and adjust your fasting period if necessary. Some days might require a shorter fasting window, and that's okay. The goal is a sustainable change that benefits your well-being, not a rigid program that adds stress.

Managing Energy Levels

As your body adapts to intermittent fasting, you may notice fluctuations in your energy levels. Organizing your day around your energy peaks and troughs can help. For instance, if you're more energetic in the morning, schedule demanding tasks during this time and allow for easier activities when your energy dips. This strategic approach can make the transition smoother and more manageable.

Emotional Considerations

The psychological aspect of changing eating patterns can sometimes be as challenging as the physical ones. Feelings of frustration or failure might surface if results don't appear immediately or if you struggle with adhering strictly to your intended fasting schedule. It's essential to approach intermittent fasting with a mindset that embraces flexibility and patience. Celebrate small victories and be compassionate with yourself during setbacks.

Social and Family Dynamics

Dietary changes can affect more than just the individual; they can influence family meals and social gatherings. Communicate with your family about your new eating schedule and discuss how they can support you. Find ways to engage in family activities that don't center around food during your fasting hours, or prepare meals that everyone can enjoy during your eating window to maintain that invaluable family connection.

Regular Evaluation

As days turn into weeks, take time to evaluate the effects of intermittent fasting. Are you experiencing improved sleep? Better hormonal balance? Weight management? Keep a journal to note not only your physical reactions but also any emotional insights. This ongoing evaluation will help you determine if and how you should adjust your fasting regime to better serve your health goals.

Professional Guidance

Even with ample personal research and preparation, consulting with a healthcare provider knowledgeable in both menopause and dietary interventions like intermittent fasting is advisable. They can provide personalized guidance based on your health history and current condition, ensuring your diet transition is both safe and effective.

By following these guidelines, you can embrace intermittent fasting as not just a diet, but as a sustainable lifestyle change that enhances your menopausal journey. The goal is to integrate fasting naturally into your life, respecting and listening to your body's signals, and supporting your overall health and well-being.

Debunking Common Fasting Myths and Facts

In the quest toward embracing a healthier lifestyle through intermittent fasting, it's essential to clear the fog of common myths and misconceptions that often circulate about this practice. Understanding what's true and what isn't can empower you to make informed decisions and can ease your transition into fasting, particularly during the menopause phase when your body is already dealing with hormonal upheavals. Let's address these myths with clarity and scientific insight, ensuring that your fasting journey is both effective and enjoyable.

Myth 1: Fasting Leads to Severe Hunger All Day

A common fear among beginners is the overwhelming hunger they assume will consume their fasting hours. However, what many find instead is that after the initial adaptation period, their bodies adjust. Hunger levels often decrease due to the stabilization of blood sugar and the increased production of ketone bodies, which have a natural appetite-suppressing effect. Instead of constant hunger, many report increased feelings of satiety and control over their appetite during and even beyond the fasting periods.

Myth 2: Intermittent Fasting Causes Muscle Loss

The concern that fasting leads to muscle wastage is widespread but largely unfounded when fasting is done correctly. The human body is designed to preserve muscle mass during periods of food scarcity. When you fast, growth hormone levels actually increase, which helps protect muscle tissues. Moreover, as long as you consume sufficient protein during your eating windows and engage in regular strength training, you can maintain—and even build—muscle mass during intermittent fasting.

Myth 3: Fasting Slows Down Metabolism

Many assume that intermittent fasting slows metabolism due to reduced caloric intake. In reality, short-term fasts have been shown to increase metabolic rates. This boost happens as norepinephrine—a fat-burning hormone—is released to utilize fat as an energy source. It is prolonged calorie restriction that can lead to a decrease in metabolic rate, but intermittent fasting, especially when meals are balanced, does not equate to severe calorie restriction and thus does not trigger metabolic slowdown.

Myth 4: It's Unnecessary to Pay Attention to Diet Quality

There's a misconception that if you're fasting, the quality of what you eat during your eating windows doesn't matter—as long as you stick to the fasting schedule. This couldn't be further from the truth. The benefits of intermittent fasting can be significantly enhanced by focusing on a nutrient-dense diet. Menopausal women, in particular, need to ensure they are getting enough calcium, iron, fiber, and vitamins from whole foods to support overall health. Good nutrition also helps in managing potential fasting side-effects, ensuring that your energy levels remain stable.

Myth 5: Fasting is Inappropriate for Menopausal Women

Some believe that the hormonal fluctuations during menopause make fasting risky or less effective. On the contrary, intermittent fasting can offer numerous benefits during menopause, including improved insulin sensitivity, better fat distribution, and enhanced mood and cognitive function. The key is to approach fasting softly—gradually increasing fasting windows and ensuring nutritional intake is balanced, particularly focusing on those nutrients critical for menopausal health.

Myth 6: Everyone Benefits from the Same Fasting Regime

Just as no two bodies are the same, no single fasting schedule works universally for everyone. While the 16/8 method may be popular, it might not suit everyone, especially during menopause when sensitivity to changes can be heightened. Listening to your body's signals and adjusting the fasting type, durations, and eating windows accordingly is essential for realizing the full benefits of intermittent fasting tailored to individual needs and health status.

Myth 7: Fasting Automatically Results in Nutrient Deficiency

Provided that your eating windows consist of diverse, balanced, and nutrient-dense foods, intermittent fasting should not lead to deficiencies. Planning meals to include a variety of food groups—fruits, vegetables, proteins, and fats—ensures that you receive the essential vitamins and minerals. Regular monitoring and potentially supplementing based on a healthcare provider's advice can help prevent any nutritional gaps.

Wrapping Up the Facts

Armed with factual knowledge and debunked myths, initiating and sustaining an intermittent fasting regimen can become a less daunting and more enlightening journey. As you consider incorporating fasting into your lifestyle, especially during menopause, remember that personalized adaptation and a focus on overall well-being can guide your decisions. Intermittent fasting isn't just a dietary choice; it's a path towards reclaiming control over your health, enhancing your quality of life, and nurturing your body through a period of significant change.

INCORPORATING FASTING INTO DAILY LIFE

Incorporating intermittent fasting into daily life can seem daunting at first, especially amid the hormonal shifts and changes that accompany menopause. However, with the right approach, it can seamlessly blend into your routine, enhancing your health without overwhelming your day-to-day life. The key lies in customizing the practice to fit your personal lifestyle, responsibilities, and health goals. Here we explore how to integrate fasting into your life comprehensively and sustainably.

Start Small and Scale Gradually

The beauty of intermittent fasting lies in its flexibility; there's no need to dive into strict regimens immediately. Begin with smaller fasting windows and allow your body and schedule to adjust naturally. For instance, if typically breakfast is at 7 AM, consider pushing it to 8 AM or 9 AM initially, and similarly, pull dinner time a bit earlier. These small adjustments can dramatically reduce the stress of adaptation.

Align Fasting with Natural Rhythms

Pay attention to your body's natural rhythms and energy cycles. Some individuals feel more energetic and clear-headed in the morning, making it simpler to skip breakfast and fast until noon. Others might find that an early dinner and fasting overnight suits them better. Listen to your body's responses and tailor your fasting schedule accordingly, aligning it with your most energetic periods to capitalize on natural feelings of satiety and alertness.

Integrate with Social and Family Activities

Fasting shouldn't isolate you or complicate your social life. Plan your eating windows around typical family meals or social gatherings. This way, you can partake in communal eating, which is both a joyous and important aspect of social interactions. You can still engage in activities during fasting times—like going for walks or attending events—balancing both social pleasure and your fasting commitments without feeling left out.

Utilize Technology

Leverage technology to ease your fasting journey. Several apps not only track fasting and eating windows but also provide reminders and motivational support. These tools can help manage your schedule, remind you when fasting windows close, and keep a log of your progress, making the practice manageable alongside a busy lifestyle.

Prepare for Hunger Pangs

During the initial stages of fasting, you may experience hunger pangs. Prepare for these moments by planning activities that can divert your attention—such as reading, meditating, or engaging in light exercises like yoga. Drinking plenty of water, herbal teas, or even coffee without additives can also help manage hunger without breaking your fast.

Educate Yourself Continuously

Understanding the science behind intermittent fasting strengthens your commitment and helps adapt the practice as part of a healthy lifestyle. The more informed you are, the better equipped you will be to handle challenges and make adjustments. Reading up on the latest research can provide new insights and motivation, making your fasting journey an evolving process of learning and growth.

Listen to Your Body

Always be attentive to how your body reacts to changes in your fasting regimen. If you experience prolonged fatigue, mood swings, or other negative symptoms, reassess your approach. Maybe your fasting windows need adjusting, or perhaps your intake during eating periods needs more balance. Continuous tuning and adapting are crucial, especially under the flux of menopause.

Keep a Journal

Keeping a journal provides insights into both your physical and emotional responses to fasting. Record times of your fasting, types of food consumed, your feelings, and any physical symptoms. This log can serve as a useful reference to track what works best for you and help identify patterns that lead to a more successful fasting experience.

Seek Support

Community support is invaluable, especially when making significant lifestyle changes. Join online groups, forums, or local communities that focus on intermittent fasting. Sharing experiences, challenges, and successes with others who are on a similar path can provide encouragement, accountability, and new ideas, improving your chances of sustaining your fasting routine.

Respect Your Progress

Remember, every step you take towards incorporating fasting into your life is progress. There may be days when things don't go as planned, but rather than feeling discouraged, use these moments as learning opportunities. Celebrate the days when you successfully follow through, and gently steer yourself back on track on tougher days.

By appreciating your unique journey and adapting intermittent fasting to fit into your personal and social lifestyle, you can effectively make it a natural part of your routine. It's not just about health benefits; it's about creating a flexible, enjoyable lifestyle that acknowledges and respects your body's needs during menopause and beyond.

3. THE BASICS OF ANTI-INFLAMMATORY EATING

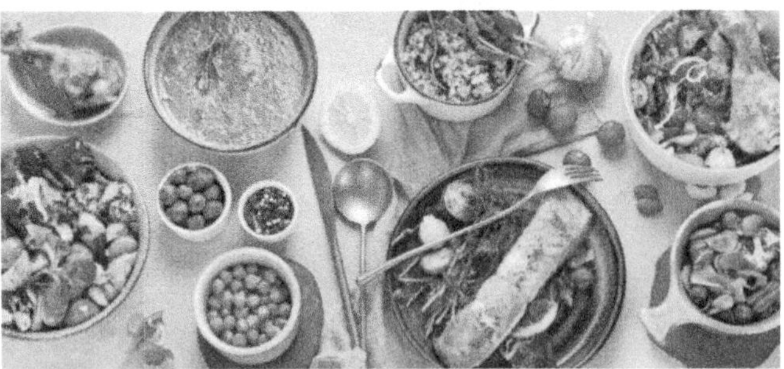

As we gracefully navigate the waves of menopause, the impact of our diet becomes increasingly evident—not just on our waistlines but on our overall health and well-being. Entering the realm of anti-inflammatory eating is akin to turning the key in a lock that opens the doors to enhanced health, particularly during this pivotal phase of life. This chapter delves into the core principles of anti-inflammatory eating, a vital component of your journey with the Galveston Diet, aimed at easing menopausal symptoms and reinvigorating your body.
Inflammation is the body's natural response to protect itself against harm, but when it becomes chronic, it can lead to various health issues, some of which are exacerbated during menopause. Persistent inflammation has been linked to an increased risk of heart disease, diabetes, and arthritis, not to mention its impact on daily discomforts such as bloating, fatigue, and mood swings. Therefore, addressing inflammation through diet can significantly alter your menopausal experience, turning what could be years of struggle into a time of revitalization.

The concept of an anti-inflammatory diet isn't just about removing certain foods from your plate; it's about replenishing your body with foods that are lush in nutrients, rich in colors, and abundant in life-giving energy. It's about creating meals that not only delight your palate but also soothe and heal your body. You will learn to embrace a bounty of vegetables, lean proteins, whole grains, and fats that heal—foods that work in harmony to restore hormonal balance and reduce inflammatory responses.

Imagine starting your day with a breakfast that doesn't just fill you but fuels you, diminishing the joint stiffness and reducing the swelling often felt during the early hours. Envision preparing a dinner that not only brings your family together but also brings comfort and relief to your body, nurturing it with every bite.

This approach is not about stringent restrictions or overwhelming choices; it's about making thoughtful, informed decisions that lead to a healthier, more vibrant you. By the end of this chapter, you will be equipped not only with the knowledge of why anti-inflammatory foods are crucial during menopause but also with practical ways to incorporate these healing foods into your daily routine, ensuring that each meal brings you closer to balance and wellness.

THE SIGNIFICANCE OF INFLAMMATION DURING MENOPAUSE

Understanding the intricate relationship between inflammation and menopause is a bit like piecing together a complex puzzle. Each piece represents a different aspect of your physical health affected by menopause, and inflammation is the backdrop influencing all other pieces.

During menopause, many women find that their bodies seem to rebel in ways that are both uncomfortable and unexpected. You might wake up one morning feeling achy for no apparent reason or suddenly find yourself wrestling with bouts of digestive discomfort. It's not uncommon to face an array of symptoms that, at first glance, seem unrelated to menopause. However, underlying many of these disturbances is a persistent, low-grade inflammation, an unwelcome guest that can wreak havoc in your body during these years.

In medical terms, inflammation is a natural process used by your body to protect against diseases and heal itself. When your body senses a threat, it responds by activating your immune system to dispatch white blood cells and chemical messengers to the affected areas. This works great when you're young and your body's responses are accurate. However, as estrogen levels fluctuate and eventually decrease during menopause, your body's inflammatory response can go into overdrive and become less efficient. This misfire tends to prolong the inflammatory process, leading to chronic inflammation.

Chronic inflammation has been associated with an array of health conditions that often manifest more prominently during menopause, such as joint pain, weight gain, increased risk of heart disease, and a challenged immune system. Importantly, it's not just physical discomfort that inflammation contributes to; it has significant impacts on your mental and emotional health as well, evidenced by increased episodes of anxiety and depressive moods, which are not uncommon during menopause.

So, why does inflammation become more of a player during these years? The clue lies in the hormonal orchestra that is now changing its tune. Estrogen, particularly, plays an anti-inflammatory role in your body. It works by moderating the production and effectiveness of endocrine factors involved in inflammatory processes. As menopause progresses and the levels of estrogen fluctuate and decline, this anti-inflammatory influence wanes, leading to an increase in inflammatory markers commonly seen in menopausal women.

Addressing these markers through an anti-inflammatory diet is more than just managing symptoms; it's about creating an internal environment that supports health and vitality. This diet focuses on foods known to combat inflammation, while steering clear of those that can trigger or exacerbate it.

Imagine your diet as a garden. What you want to grow are lush, vibrant plants (or in this case, cells and organs functioning at their best). To achieve this vibrant garden, you need to nurture it with water and sunlight while keeping out weeds (inflammatory foods) and pests (toxins and stress) which can overrun your beautiful space. Just like gardening, implementing an anti-inflammatory diet requires understanding what nourishes your body and what harms it.

Common inflammatory foods that are advisable to limit or avoid include refined sugars and carbohydrates, which can cause insulin spikes and weight gain; trans fats found in many fried and processed foods; and excessive alcohol. Instead, your dietary focus during menopause should lean heavily towards whole, unprocessed foods—colorful fruits and vegetables, lean proteins, and healthy fats. These foods are not only rich in nutrients but also contain antioxidants and phytochemicals that help combat inflammation.

Beyond the basics of choosing the right foods, it's also crucial to tailor your consumption patterns to what suits your body best during menopause. This isn't a one-size-fits-all journey. Some women might find that dairy products exacerbate their symptoms, while others might discover a new sensitivity to gluten. Tracking how your body responds to different foods and adjusting your diet accordingly can profoundly affect how you manage inflammation and, by extension, how you experience menopause.

This individual approach is significant because inflammation isn't just a general threat; it's a highly personal one that varies dramatically from one woman to another. The subtlety lies in forging a path that works precisely for you—an eating strategy that respects and responds to your body's changing needs.

Effective management of inflammation throughout menopause is pivotal not just for alleviating immediate discomfort but for preventing long-term health complications. By making informed dietary choices, you set the stage for a healthier menopausal transition, improving your quality of life and well-being.

In sum, tackling inflammation with a strategic diet during menopause is empowering. It returns a measure of control to you, allowing you to actively influence how you feel each day. This empowerment is what the Galveston Diet aims to provide—guidelines backed by science, personalized to suit your unique journey through menopause. As we move forward, the focus will shift to not just understanding but practically integrating anti-inflammatory eating into your lifestyle, ensuring that each meal is a step towards balancing your body's inflammatory response and enhancing your overall health.

Anti-Inflammatory Foods to Incorporate

Navigating through menopause is often akin to sailing through shifting seas. The ebb and flow of hormonal changes can leave you feeling unsteady. What if you could find an anchor in your diet, something to help stabilize and soothe those swells? Turning to anti-inflammatory foods is that stabilizing force, a way to calm the internal storms of menopause, reducing inflammation and fostering better overall health.

The journey into anti-inflammatory eating doesn't begin with a list of strict do's and don'ts—rather, it starts with an understanding and appreciation of foods that nourish and heal. These are foods packed with nutrients that naturally curb inflammatory responses in the body, promoting healing and comfort. As you embark on this journey, imagine each meal as a vibrant palette of colors and textures, each component not just pleasing to the palate but also profoundly beneficial to your body.

Fruits and vegetables are the cornerstone of any anti-inflammatory diet. Rich in antioxidants, vitamins, and minerals, they help fortify the body against oxidative stress, a key player in inflammation. Berries, for instance, with their deep hues of red, blue, and purple, aren't just delightful to look at—they're also packed with antioxidants like quercetin and anthocyanins. Picture starting your day with a bowl of mixed berries, a simple yet powerful way to introduce anti-inflammatory agents into your system from the get-go.

Leafy greens, such as spinach, kale, and Swiss chard, are loaded with vitamins A, C, and K and flavonoids that play crucial roles in reducing inflammation. Integrating these into your diet through a delicious stir-fry or a fresh salad can make a difference in how you feel. Imagine the crunch of kale in your mouth, it's not just a texture, it's a burst of anti-inflammatory goodness.

Another pivotal chapter in the anti-inflammatory diet book is the inclusion of healthy fats. These are not the villains we once thought them to be; instead, they are essential allies. Omega-3 fatty acids, which are abundantly found in fish like salmon, mackerel, and sardines, are known for their inflammation-reducing capabilities. Visualize enjoying a piece of grilled salmon, its flavors rich, knowing that with every bite, you are feeding your body something good, something essential.

Alongside omega-3s, nuts and seeds like almonds, walnuts, flaxseeds, and chia seeds are valuable additions to your diet. They not only add a nutty crunch to your meals but bring with them a generous helping of anti-inflammatory benefits, thanks to their high content of healthy fats and fiber. Adding a handful of these to a smoothie or sprinkling them over a salad can transform an ordinary meal into an anti-inflammatory powerhouse.

Spices and herbs not only add flavors to your dishes but can significantly dial down inflammation. Turmeric, with its active compound curcumin, has been extensively studied for its potent anti-inflammatory properties and is easy to incorporate into your cooking. Imagine sprinkling golden turmeric on your vegetables or blending it into a smoothie, each spoonful a strike against inflammation. Similarly, ginger, garlic, and cinnamon, each with their unique qualities, can make your meals not only tastier but healthier.

Beyond what is often highlighted in typical dietary guides, certain beverages can also play an role in reducing inflammation. Green tea, for example, is famed not just for its ability to energize but also for its catechins, antioxidant compounds that effectively fight inflammation and may even aid in weight management. Imagine sipping a warm cup of green tea, each gulp infusing your body with healing compounds.

Integrating these foods into your daily regimen doesn't require drastic changes—start small. Maybe introduce a new vegetable or fruit each week, experiment with fish varieties, or explore flavors with spices and herbs you haven't used before. Each small step is a leap towards healing.

Perhaps the true beauty of an anti-inflammatory diet lies not just in the foods you eat, but in the life-changing impacts these foods have. Each ingredient carries not just flavor but the potential for a transformed bodily response—less pain, more comfort, and a smoother journey through menopause.

Remember, embracing anti-inflammatory foods is less about adhering to a rigid diet and more about making a lifestyle shift—a commitment to nourish your body with every meal. While this chapter closes here, the journey towards a healthful, vibrant life continues, with each food choice paving the way towards a healthier menopause experience. Every meal is a new opportunity to take control, to soothe, and to heal.

Foods to Eliminate

In the journey toward managing menopause symptoms through diet, it becomes equally crucial to know what to remove from your plate as it is to understand what to add. As we explore the realm of anti-inflammatory eating, recognizing the foods that could potentially exacerbate inflammation leads us to make wiser choices for our meals, thus mitigating menopausal discomfort and promoting overall well-being.

The foods that generally spearhead inflammation are often those that are hardest to give up, not only because they might be habitual but because they are so prevalent in our food supply. These include heavily processed foods, sugary treats, and certain types of fat which, while offering momentary gratification, can cause long-term disruptions in the way your body naturally fights inflammation.

Think of your body as a finely tuned instrument. Each wrong input—like certain types of food—can detune this instrument. The first group we'll discuss is processed sugars. Picture your favorite cookies, cakes, or soft drinks—delicious, yes, but they could be contributing to a higher level of inflammation in your body. Processed sugars trigger the release of cytokines, inflammatory messenger molecules, which can lead to a cascade of unwanted inflammatory responses. They also contribute to weight gain, which is a common challenge during menopause and which, in itself, promotes inflammation.

Next, consider the role of refined carbohydrates found in products like white bread, pastries, and various snacks. These are high glycemic index foods that cause spikes in your blood sugar and insulin levels, fostering an environment that can escalate inflammatory processes. Like a sugar rush that ends with a crash, refined carbs provide an immediate energy boost followed by an inevitable depletion of energy, complicating your body's inflammatory response.

Trans fats are another inflammatory culprit to consider eliminating. Often hidden in deep-fried foods, fast food, and some margarines, trans fats are known for increasing harmful LDL cholesterol while lowering beneficial HDL cholesterol, fostering inflammation, obesity, and resistance to insulin. Each of these factors plays a significant role in how menopausal symptoms manifest and compound.

Partially hydrogenated oils, found in some processed and packaged foods, are primary sources of trans fats. Imagine these oils as 'wolves in sheep's clothing', where they appear innocent in many popular snack foods but covertly contribute to inflammation and deteriorating heart health.

Further down the path of inflammatory foods are excessive amounts of omega-6 fatty acids. While omega-6s are essential fats that the body cannot produce on its own, an imbalance between omega-6 and omega-3 fatty acids can lead to inflammation. Typical western diets tend to be high in omega-6 fatty acids due to the common use of vegetable oils like corn, soybean, and sunflower oil in cooking and processed foods. Adjusting this balance by reducing omega-6 intake and increasing omega-3 rich foods like flaxseeds, walnuts, and fatty fish can provide considerable benefits in managing inflammation.

Alcohol, in moderation, might offer some health benefits, particularly red wine, which is known for containing resveratrol, a compound that has potential anti-inflammatory properties. However, excessive alcohol consumption is decidedly pro-inflammatory.

It impairs organ functions and disrupts the immune system, which can exacerbate inflammatory responses, not to mention its effects on disrupting sleep patterns—already a significant challenge during menopause.

Lastly, artificial additives found in numerous processed foods may also contribute to inflammation. These include artificial sweeteners and flavors and preservatives that ensure longer shelf lives but may be detrimental to body health when consumed frequently. When ingested, these compounds can trigger immune responses which can further lead to or exacerbate inflammation.

Eliminating or significantly reducing these foods from your diet isn't just about depriving yourself of guilty pleasures; it's about re-tuning your body to perform its symphony harmoniously. It's about replacing the momentary satisfaction of inflammatory foods with lasting comfort and improved health.

Transitioning away from these foods to more wholesome, anti-inflammatory options doesn't have to feel like a sacrifice. It's an empowering lifestyle adjustment that, while challenging, reaps significant rewards. Each step you take away from inflammatory foods and toward nourishing alternatives is a step toward reclaiming control over your health and your menopause experience.

In making these adjustments, be patient with yourself. Dietary changes, especially profound ones, require time to integrate and yield visible results. Encourage yourself by focusing on the variety and richness of the foods you can enjoy and the benefits they offer, rather than those you are avoiding. This positive approach not only makes the transition smoother but also more fulfilling and sustainable in the long run.

Setting Up an Anti-Inflammatory Kitchen

Embarking on a journey towards an anti-inflammatory lifestyle begins right in the heart of your home: the kitchen. This space, where meals are prepared and often shared, can transform into your personal wellness haven, a place where every tool and ingredient serves a purpose toward better health. Setting up your kitchen strategically not only supports your anti-inflammatory diet but also makes the process of cooking and meal preparation an act of self-care.

Visualize your kitchen right now. Perhaps it's filled with gadgets you hardly use or foods that don't necessarily serve your new health goals. Now, imagine it transformed: streamlined counters with foods rich in nutrients, cabinets stocked with health-supporting herbs and spices, and a refrigerator brimming with vibrant fruits and vegetables. This kitchen doesn't just facilitate cooking; it promotes a lifestyle.

The first step in this transformation is clearing the clutter. This means going through every cabinet and drawer and removing processed foods that sabotage your anti-inflammatory intentions. These could be items high in refined sugars, unhealthy fats, and additives—foods that might be convenient but likely fuel inflammation in the body. Removing these not only clears space but also removes temptation, making it easier to commit to healthier eating habits.

Next, prioritize organization. Having a well-organized kitchen saves time and reduces stress, making the cooking process more enjoyable. Invest in clear containers to store whole grains, nuts, and seeds. Not only do these containers keep ingredients fresh, but they also give you clear visual access to all your healthy options, encouraging their use. Consider placing these items at eye level in your pantry or on your countertop, where they are easily accessible and thus more likely to be used.

The right tools can also make all the difference. Equip your kitchen with high-quality kitchenware that makes preparing fruits, vegetables, and lean meats simpler and more efficient. A good set of knives, cutting boards for different food types (to avoid cross-contamination), non-stick ceramic or cast-iron pans, and a powerful blender for smoothies and soups can enhance your meal prep experience. These tools make it easier to prepare meals from scratch, which is a cornerstone of eating well during menopause.

Incorporating plenty of anti-inflammatory herbs and spices is crucial, so create a dedicated space for these powerful tools. Turmeric, ginger, garlic, and cinnamon should be staples in your arsenal, easily reachable when cooking. Storing them properly to maintain their potency is key—cool, dark places in airtight containers work best. With these at your fingertips, you can easily add an anti-inflammatory boost to any dish.

Stocking up on anti-inflammatory staples is next. Fill your pantry with whole grains like quinoa, barley, and oats. Ensure your refrigerator is filled with leafy greens, nuts, seeds, and fatty fish, ensuring they are the first things you see when you open the door. Opt for fresh whenever possible, but remember that frozen vegetables and fruits can be just as nutritious and are great to have on hand for quick meals.

Hydration plays a significant role in reducing inflammation as well, so setting up a hydration station in your kitchen can serve as a constant reminder to drink water throughout the day. A simple pitcher filled with filtered water, perhaps infused with anti-inflammatory cucumber or lemon, can be both refreshing and health-promoting.

As you revamp your kitchen, pay attention to how your space makes you feel. Incorporating elements that bring joy and calm can encourage a positive relationship with cooking and eating. Maybe it's a vase of fresh flowers, some inspiring art on the walls, or even just ensuring you have good lighting and a clean, welcoming space.

Equally important is how you approach eating. Setting up a pleasant dining area that invites you to enjoy your meals without distraction can change your relationship with food. Eating slowly and mindfully can not only improve digestion but can also help you better integrate your dietary changes into your lifestyle.

Remember, the goal of configuring your kitchen for anti-inflammatory eating isn't just about following a diet—it's about crafting a lifestyle that naturally promotes health and well-being. Each step in this setup is a piece in the puzzle of your health journey, each tool and ingredient a building block in your path to wellness. As this chapter of your journey unfolds, you'll find that a well-prepared kitchen environment empowers you to make choices that support your menopausal health goals, making each meal a step towards a vibrant, energized life.

4.Foundational Concepts of The Galveston Diet

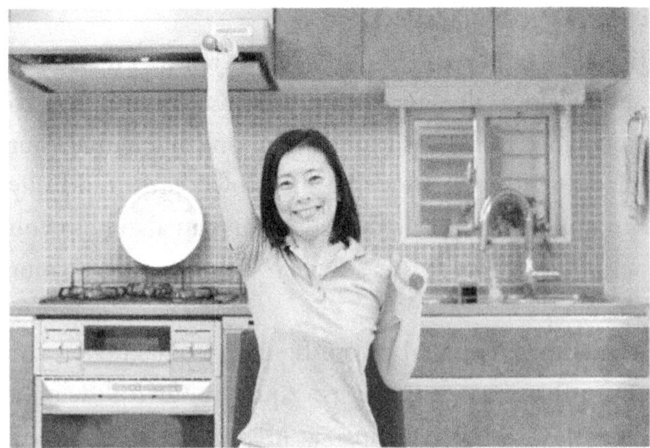

As we explore the foundational concepts of the Galveston Diet, we delve into a strategy that is more than just dietary change; it's a transformative lifestyle designed specifically for the unique needs of menopausal women. This diet isn't about mere weight loss or restricting pleasures; it's about rekindling a harmonious relationship between your body and the foods you consume.

Imagine entering a phase of your life where your body suddenly seems to be rewriting the rules. During menopause, hormonal fluctuations can lead to increased inflammation and shifts in metabolism, making traditional diets less effective or even counterproductive. That's where the Galveston Diet comes into play. It precisely adjusts your intake of macronutrients – proteins, fats, and carbohydrates – to support hormonal balance and reduce inflammation, two critical factors in menopausal health.

Here's a scenario many of us can relate to: you're following a meal plan that was once effective but now seems to lead nowhere. This common frustration during menopause is often due to not addressing the root of the problem—hormonal imbalance and inflammation. By focusing on high-quality proteins and healthy fats, the Galveston Diet doesn't just fill you up; it nourishes your body and optimizes your metabolic health. Proteins are the building blocks for your body's repair systems, and healthy fats are vital for hormonal balance.

Moreover, don't overlook the role of carbohydrates and dietary fiber. While it's easy to demonize carbs in our diet culture, the Galveston Diet teaches us to choose wisely—focusing on fiber-rich vegetables and whole grains that can help stabilize blood sugar levels and support digestive health, without causing inflammation.

Water, often underestimated in its importance, is highlighted in its role as a carrier of nutrients and a key element in maintaining cellular health and detoxification.

Adopting the Galveston Diet isn't just about what we eliminate but about creating a vibrant, varied plate that caters to deeper nutritional needs—empowering your body to navigate through menopause with vitality and grace. This thoughtful approach to eating can reignite your body's innate ability to find balance, promoting a healthier, more vibrant you as you move through this chapter of your life.

Adjusting Macronutrients for Menopause

As menopause approaches, it often arrives not with a whisper, but with a cacophony of hormonal fluctuations that redefine the way our bodies manage energy, metabolism, and overall wellness. One of the most profound shifts occurs in how our bodies respond to macronutrients—the proteins, fats, and carbohydrates that are the cornerstone of our diets.

Understanding Macronutrient Needs During Menopause

Let's start by rethinking proteins, fats, and carbohydrates not just as fuel but as dynamic components interacting with our shifting hormonal landscape. Menopause introduces a significant decrease in estrogen levels, a hormone that, among many roles, helps regulate metabolism and body weight. What many do not realize is that this hormonal change alters the way our body processes each macronutrient, demanding a nuanced approach to our plates.

The Role of Protein: More Than Just Muscle

The importance of protein elevates as we age, especially during menopause. Proteins are essential for maintaining muscle mass, which naturally tends to decrease in our later years. Lesser muscle mass is synonymous with a slower metabolism, which can contribute to weight gain—a common concern among menopausal women.

But it's not simply about quantity; it's the quality of protein that also counts. Incorporating a variety of high-quality proteins, such as lean meats, fish rich in omega-3 fatty acids, legumes, and tofu helps ensure a spectrum of essential amino acids that support overall body functions. These proteins act as building blocks for enzymes and hormones, playing a pivotal role in maintaining hormonal balance and muscle integrity.

Healthy Fats: Nurturing Hormonal Harmony

As the production of key hormones drops, the right kinds of dietary fats can become powerful allies. Healthy fats, particularly those rich in omega-3 and omega-6 fatty acids, are fundamental in creating a favorable environment for hormonal equilibrium. These fats are not just crucial for absorption of fat-soluble vitamins like A, D, E, and K but are also vital in the production of hormones.

Avocados, nuts, seeds, and fatty fish are potent sources of these beneficial fats. They contribute to reducing inflammation—which tends to increase during menopause—and aid in the modulation of metabolic health. The strategic adjustment isn't just adding fats indiscriminately, but choosing sources that contribute to health without exacerbating menopausal symptoms like weight gain.

Rethinking Carbohydrates: Quality Over Quantity

Carbohydrates often bear the brunt of diet discussions, particularly around issues of weight gain. During menopause, sensitivity to carbohydrates can increase, leading to heightened blood sugar spikes and subsequent crashes. This doesn't mean eliminating carbohydrates altogether but rather choosing types that have a minimal impact on blood sugar.

Focusing on fiber-rich carbohydrates—think vegetables, whole grains, and legumes—ensures that you gain the nutritional benefits of these foods without the steep spikes in insulin. Such carbohydrates help maintain a feeling of fullness, reduce cravings, and support digestive health, which can sometimes be compromised during menopause.

Dietary Fiber: The Unsung Hero

While technically not a macronutrient, dietary fiber deserves a special mention for its role in menopausal health management. Fiber aids in digestion, helps regulate blood sugar levels, and can even bind to excess hormones and remove them from the body. Foods high in fiber, such as fruits, vegetables, and whole grains, should be staples in the menopausal diet not only for their nutrient density but for their role in maintaining stable energy levels and supporting metabolic health.

Water: Supporting Metabolic Processes

Water, though not a macronutrient, dramatically influences how macronutrients are processed in the body. Hydration becomes increasingly crucial as we age, as water helps manage body temperature (think hot flashes), facilitates digestion, and aids in the transport of nutrients. Menopausal women should aim to increase their water intake to support these essential bodily functions.

Adjusting Your Plate

Adjusting the macronutrient composition of your meals requires a thoughtful balance that respects your body's changing needs. A plate during menopause might look different—richer in proteins and healthy fats, careful with carbohydrates, and abundant in fiber-rich plants. This doesn't mean a restrictive diet but a thoughtful one, curated to support your body through the transitions it's experiencing.

Embracing the Changes

Understanding and adjusting to your body's new needs is a profound way to support yourself during menopause. By modifying your intake of macronutrients to better align with your body's current status, you create a dietary strategy that not only addresses weight management but also enhances your overall well-being. Each meal becomes an opportunity to nourish your body deeply and holistically, turning food into an ally during this significant life transition.

By harnessing the power of macronutrients thoughtfully and deliberately, you can mitigate many of the physical challenges posed by menopause. The goal is to transform your diet into one that supports and sustains your health through menopause and beyond. This journey is as much about what you eat as it is about relearning and listening to your body's cues, ensuring that every bite moves you toward hormonal balance and vibrant health.

Prioritizing High-Quality Proteins and Healthy Fats

In the journey through menopause, the foods we choose become not just fuel but vital allies in managing the complex cascade of bodily changes. Among these choices, high-quality proteins and healthy fats stand out as cornerstones of the Galveston Diet, playing pivotal roles in maintaining hormonal equilibrium and overall health during this transformative period.

High-Quality Proteins: Building Blocks for a Healthier Menopause

Protein is crucial in any diet, but its importance becomes particularly pronounced during menopause. It's not just about combating muscle loss that naturally occurs with age; it's also about supporting the structural integrity of cells and facilitating the optimal functioning of enzymes and hormones. High-quality proteins contain all the essential amino acids our bodies need but can't produce independently.

Sources like lean meats, fish, dairy, and legumes not only provide these essential amino acids but also contain other vital nutrients beneficial during menopause, such as iron, which can help combat the fatigue often reported in menopausal women. Moreover, fish such as salmon, mackerel, and sardines are rich in omega-3 fatty acids, known for their anti-inflammatory properties, which are crucial since inflammation can increase during menopause.

Yet, not all proteins are created equal. The distinction of 'high-quality' refers to proteins that are easily absorbed and utilized by the body, a vital aspect, particularly when the digestive system might also be experiencing changes due to menopause. Integrating varied protein sources ensures a broad spectrum of nutritional benefits. For instance, combining plant-based proteins such as beans and rice can provide a complete amino acid profile similar to that found in meats.

Healthy Fats: More Than Just Calories

The role of fats in the diet has often been misunderstood, shadowed by the stigma of weight gain. However, healthy fats, particularly mono- and polyunsaturated fats, are crucial during menopause for their role in hormone production and regulation. These fats are not merely a source of energy but are vital components of cell membranes, ensuring fluidity and functionality.

In the context of menopause, fats are doubly important. They aid in the absorption of fat-soluble vitamins—Vitamins A, D, E, and K—which support bone health, immune function, and cellular repair processes that are vital during menopause. Moreover, the anti-inflammatory properties of omega-3 fatty acids can help manage and reduce systemic inflammation that often accompanies this stage, hence reducing instances of joint pain, skin changes, and other inflammatory symptoms.

Sources like avocados, nuts, seeds, and olive oil not only enhance the absorption of nutrients from other foods but also provide antioxidants that combat oxidative stress, another common issue during menopause that accelerates aging and increases the risk of chronic diseases.

The Synergistic Effects of Proteins and Fats

When proteins and fats are combined correctly in the diet, they can help stabilize blood sugar levels by slowing down carbohydrate absorption and enhancing satiety. This is particularly beneficial during menopause, a time when many women struggle with weight gain due to hormonal changes and a naturally declining metabolic rate.

Consider, for instance, a meal that combines grilled salmon (rich in protein and omega-3 fatty acids) with a side of avocado salad (packed with fiber and mono-unsaturated fats). This meal not only satisfies but also supports hormonal balance, promotes cardiovascular health, and combats inflammation.

Strategic Integration into Your Diet

Embracing a diet high in quality proteins and healthy fats doesn't necessarily require a drastic overhaul of eating habits, but rather a mindful modification. It's about making choices that align with metabolic and hormonal needs. Small, consistent changes can lead to sustainable health benefits. For example, switching from butter to olive oil for cooking, choosing nuts or a piece of fruit rather than chips for a snack, or opting for lean poultry instead of red meat can collectively enhance your diet's nutritional profile without feeling restrictive.

Tuning into Your Body's Signals

Every woman's experience of menopause is unique, and so too should be her dietary approach. It's imperative to listen to your body and adjust your intake of proteins and fats according to how you feel. Some might find certain foods exacerbate symptoms like bloating or indigestion—the key is to identify these responses and tailor your diet accordingly.

Maintaining a nutrient-rich diet that prioritizes high-quality proteins and healthy fats can transform the menopausal experience from a time of difficulty to a stage of empowerment. By understanding and implementing these nutritional strategies, you equip your body with the tools it needs to transition through menopause smoothly and healthily. This approach isn't just about managing symptoms but about fostering a way of life that embraces change with strength, resilience, and vitality. Through thoughtful dietary choices, the journey through menopause can become a path to rediscovery and rejuvenation, highlighting this stage of life not as an end but a profound new beginning.

Insights into Carbohydrates and Dietary Fiber

Amidst the myriad changes that occur during menopause, altering your dietary intake of carbohydrates and boosting dietary fiber can have a profound impact on how you feel and function. Understanding the strategic role of these nutritional components offers a way to mitigate some of the challenging symptoms associated with menopause while promoting long-term health.

The Dual Role of Carbohydrates

Carbohydrates often get a bad rap in diet culture, primarily due to their association with weight gain and metabolic disturbances. However, not all carbohydrates exert the same effects on the body. Their impact pivots significantly on their type—simple versus complex—and their fiber content.

During menopause, the body's insulin sensitivity may decrease, a development that calls for a nuanced approach to carbohydrate consumption. Simple carbohydrates, including sugars and refined flours, are quickly broken down by the body, leading to rapid spikes in blood sugar levels followed by equally swift crashes. These spikes and crashes can exacerbate menopause symptoms such as mood swings, fatigue, and even hot flashes.

In contrast, complex carbohydrates like whole grains, legumes, and most vegetables break down slower, resulting in a more gradual rise in blood sugar levels. This steadiness can help manage energy levels more effectively throughout the day, reducing fatigue and preventing the irritability associated with sugar crashes.

Leveraging Dietary Fiber for Menopausal Health

Dietary fiber is a type of carbohydrate that the body can't digest. Found in plant foods, fiber comes in two forms: soluble and insoluble. Soluble fiber dissolves in water to form a gel-like material, which can help lower blood cholesterol and glucose levels. Insoluble fiber, on the other hand, helps bulk up stool and is beneficial for those who struggle with constipation, a common issue in menopausal women.

Increasing fiber intake can have several benefits during menopause. Firstly, it enhances feelings of fullness after meals, which can help control weight by reducing the tendency to snack excessively. Additionally, fiber supports digestive health and can ease some of the gastrointestinal distress associated with hormonal changes.

The broader effects of a high-fiber diet extend beyond digestion. Fiber helps regulate the body's use of sugars, keeping hunger and blood sugar in check. It's also been noted to play a role in reducing systemic inflammation—a notable benefit, considering that increased inflammation is linked to many chronic diseases, as well as heightened menopause symptoms.

Strategic Choices in Carbohydrate Selection

Choosing the right types of carbohydrates is key. Integrating a variety of whole grains like quinoa, barley, and oats—not only diversifies your diet but also provides a substantive base of minerals, vitamins, and antioxidants. Vegetables, particularly leafy greens and those rich in color (like bell peppers and carrots), offer a good mix of carbohydrates and fiber, plus they are laden with phytonutrients that support overall health.

Beans and legumes represent another excellent source of both complex carbohydrates and fiber. They're also an excellent alternative protein source, which can be particularly useful for those looking to reduce their meat consumption.

Practical Tips for Incorporating Healthy Carbohydrates and Fibers

To start, consider replacing white bread, rice, and pasta with their whole-grain counterparts. Experiment with fiber-rich grains like bulgur, farro, or millet, which not only enrich the diet but can also introduce new textures and flavors to meals. Aim to include a vegetable at every meal—not just dinner—and think about fruits as a source of natural sweetness that also brings fiber and key nutrients to the table.

Snacking also offers a prime opportunity to increase fiber intake. Opt for raw veggies, nuts, seeds, or whole-grain crackers—choices that provide a nutritious kick without the empty calories associated with many processed snacks. Moreover, beginning your day with a high-fiber breakfast, such as a bowl of oatmeal topped with berries or chia seeds, can help maintain steady blood sugar levels throughout the day.

Tuning into Your Body's Responses

No one dietary approach fits all, especially during the menopausal transition. Pay attention to how your body responds to changes in your diet. Some might find that certain fibrous foods cause bloating or gas—adjustments might be necessary as your digestive system adapts. Monitoring how your symptoms correlate with dietary changes can be incredibly insightful and empower you to make adjustments that genuinely enhance your well-being.

Embracing a Holistic Approach

Incorporating the right balance of carbohydrates and dietary fiber into your diet during menopause is not just about reducing symptoms but improving your overall quality of life. These dietary adjustments can stabilize your energy levels, support hormonal balance, and foster a stronger, more resilient body equipped to handle the changes menopause brings.

As we navigate these transitions, remember that your diet is powerful not only in its ability to nourish but also in its capacity to heal and stabilize. By adjusting our intake of carbohydrates and emphasizing dietary fiber, we embrace a proactive stance toward our health, ensuring that our food choices support not just survival but thriving through menopause and beyond.

Water: An Essential Yet Underrated Nutrient

Water, often dubbed the elixir of life, is a crucial but frequently overlooked component of dietary health, especially during the transitional phase of menopause. This vital nutrient does far more than simply quench thirst; it plays a critical role in nearly every bodily function, including temperature regulation, nutrient transport, and waste elimination.

The Pivotal Role of Water in Menopausal Health

As women enter menopause, their bodies undergo significant hormonal changes that can impact hydration levels. Decreased estrogen levels can alter the body's ability to retain water, leading to symptoms like dry skin, fatigue, and even increased heart strain due to thicker blood consistency. These changes make maintaining proper hydration an essential component of the daily health regimen.

Hydration and Hormonal Balance

Water's role in maintaining hormonal balance is often underappreciated. Hormones are primarily transported through our bodily fluids, and dehydration can lead to their slower movement, which impacts their overall effectiveness. Proper hydration ensures that hormones such as insulin, cortisol, and even the sex hormones are adequately distributed and can function optimally. This distribution is crucial during menopause, when hormonal fluctuations are frequent and have significant physical and emotional impacts.

Water as a Thermoregulatory Agent

One of the hallmark symptoms of menopause is the hot flash, a sudden feeling of warmth that is often accompanied by sweating, redness, and even heart palpitations. These episodes are the body's attempt to cool down through perspiration. Adequate water intake helps regulate body temperature and can moderate the severity and frequency of hot flashes. Staying well-hydrated helps not only to manage these uncomfortable episodes but also to maintain overall comfort and wellness.

The Detoxifying Effects of Water

Water facilitates the removal of waste products from the body, which is carried out through sweat, urine, and feces. During menopause, the efficient removal of these waste products becomes even more important as the body adjusts to different nutritional needs and hormone levels. Ensuring ample water intake supports the liver and kidneys—organs that are pivotal in detoxification and thus directly influence menopausal health.

Cognitive Function and Emotional Well-being

Hydration also plays a crucial role in cognitive function and emotional stability. Dehydration can lead to difficulties in concentration, memory, and critical thinking. Given that menopause can already challenge emotional and cognitive health through symptoms like mood swings and memory gaps, adequate water intake becomes imperative to help mitigate these effects. Remaining hydrated helps maintain cognitive clarity and can even elevate mood, thereby improving overall well-being during menopause.

Practical Guidance for Adequate Hydration

Understanding the importance of hydration is one thing; implementing it effectively is another. Here are practical tips for incorporating more water into your daily routine:

Begin your day with water: Starting the day with a glass or two of water can kickstart your hydration and has been shown to awaken the metabolism.

Use reminders: Setting reminders on your phone or computer can prompt you to take regular water breaks, ensuring you meet your hydration goals throughout the day.

Flavor your water: If you find plain water unappealing, consider adding slices of fruits like lemon, lime, cucumber, or even a splash of juice to enhance the flavor without adding significant calories.

Eat water-rich foods: Incorporating fruits and vegetables with high water content, such as cucumbers, watermelon, oranges, and strawberries, can boost hydration.

Monitor your intake: Keeping track of how much water you drink can help develop a habit of regular water consumption. This might include marking a water bottle with times of the day by which you should have consumed a certain amount or using an app to track your intake.

Listening to Your Body

Each body is unique, and so are its hydration needs. Factors such as body size, the local climate, level of physical activity, and overall health influence how much water you should drink. While the standard recommendation is typically around eight 8-ounce glasses of water a day, listening to your body's cues, like monitoring the color of your urine, can provide personalized insight into your hydration needs. Generally, a light yellow color indicates proper hydration, while darker urine suggests a need for increased water intake.

The Integral Nature of Water in The Galveston Diet

In the Galveston Diet, water is not merely an aspect of nutrition; it is foundational to creating and sustaining hormonal balance and overall health during menopause. By prioritizing and optimizing hydration, you are taking a significant step toward enhancing your quality of life during this period of change. Embracing water as a central element of your daily routine can help smooth the menopausal transition, supporting not just physical health but also emotional and cognitive wellness.

5.Detailed Meal Planning

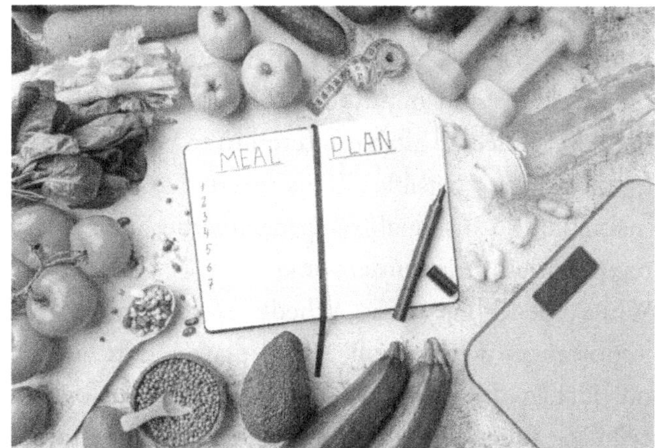

As we embark on the journey of detailed meal planning, it is imperative to recognize this as a pivotal part of managing your menopausal transition through the Galveston Diet. Crafting a meal plan isn't just about organizing what to eat and when; it's about setting a foundation for sustainable, healthful living that cherishes your body's changing needs.

Imagine your kitchen evolving into a nurturing ground for health, a place where every ingredient and meal supports your journey toward hormonal balance and weight management. Here, the spices you choose, the vegetables you chop, and the proteins you select come together not just to satisfy hunger but to nourish and revitalize your body at a cellular level.

It's Monday morning, you're standing at the kitchen counter with your meal planner. As you jot down your meals for the week, you feel a sense of control and readiness. What's key in these moments isn't merely following recipes, but understanding the why behind each food choice. For instance, knowing that a spinach-packed smoothie for breakfast injects a generous dose of iron, vital for energy levels that menopausal women often need, or that a turmeric-laced soup can act as an anti-inflammatory agent, easing joint pain and reducing flare-ups of menopausal symptoms.

Each day, by carefully selecting foods that are lush in phytoestrogens or rich in omega-3 fatty acids, you are casting a vote for a calmer, energized menopausal experience. It's not just about the sum of meals but understanding that behind each selection lies an intention, an aspect of care towards oneself.

When crafting your own 60-day meal plan, bear in mind that flexibility is your friend. Life will happen: a missed grocery shopping day, an unexpected dinner out. What matters is how you adapt—keeping the principles of anti-inflammatory and hormone-balancing foods as your guideposts.

The act of meal planning, therefore, becomes more than a routine—it transforms into an act of self-care, a testament to the importance of your health journey. Each meal planned is a step forward, a piece in the puzzle of your menopausal wellness.

Designing Your Daily Eating Schedule

Embarking on the Galveston Diet during menopause is not just about choosing the right foods; it's also about when and how you eat them. Designing your daily eating schedule is akin to painting a portrait, where each meal and snack is a stroke of color adding to your overall picture of health. This section will guide you through creating an eating schedule that harmonizes with your body's changing rhythms, enhancing your ability to manage weight, balance hormones, and maintain high energy levels throughout the day.

Let's imagine a day in your life where eating isn't just necessary, it's enjoyable and strategically planned. You wake up feeling rested, and instead of grabbing a quick, carb-heavy breakfast, you start your day with a protein-rich smoothie packed with anti-inflammatory fruits, seeds, and greens. This isn't just a breakfast; it's a deliberate choice to kickstart your metabolism and stabilize your blood sugar from the get-go.

As mid-morning approaches, instead of reaching for coffee and a pastry, you have scheduled a nutritious snack—perhaps a handful of almonds and a small, vibrant fruit. This isn't just a snack, but a tactical decision to keep your energy levels balanced and to ward off the all-too-common mid-morning slump.

Lunch is a thoughtful composition, perhaps a salad rich with leafy greens, slices of avocado, topped with grilled salmon or a hearty bean soup. This meal is aimed at maximizing your intake of omega-3 fatty acids and fiber, which are pivotal in regulating your heart health and digestive system, often affected by hormonal fluctuations during menopause.

The afternoon may present the biggest challenge, as energy levels tend to dip. This is where your foresight in scheduling comes to play. A small, nutritious snack, possibly Greek yogurt with a sprinkle of chia seeds, or a quick trail mix, can provide a sustainable energy boost. It's these small inclusions that can keep your mood and cognition buoyant as you navigate through the latter part of your day.

Dinner should be a calming, flavorful affair—maybe a stir-fry with plenty of colorful vegetables and lean protein or a piece of baked fish with a side of roasted sweet potatoes. The focus here is on light but satisfying meals that won't sit heavily but will support overnight regeneration.

And if you enjoy a small after-dinner treat, think of a portion-controlled serving of dark chocolate or a baked apple with cinnamon. These choices satisfy the sweet tooth while aligning with your anti-inflammatory goals, providing antioxidants and aiding in digestion.

Within this daily framework, also lies the principle of timing. Your last meal or snack should ideally be at least two to three hours before bedtime to support optimal sleep and digestion. It is not just about what or how much you consume, but the timing can significantly impact your sleep quality and subsequently, your overall energy levels the next day. Moreover, incorporating the principles of intermittent fasting into this schedule enriches its effectiveness. Perhaps you choose an eating window that starts with breakfast at 8 a.m. and ends with dinner at 6 p.m., allowing your digestive system a break until the next morning. This isn't mere scheduling; it's strategic eating that aligns with your body's natural rhythms, promoting better metabolism and hormone regulation.

As with any good plan, flexibility must be woven into your daily eating schedule. Life will present moments—social gatherings, family events, unexpected long meetings—that challenge this routine. The key is to navigate these with preparedness and mindfulness. Always aim to make the best choices available and return to your schedule as soon as feasible. This flexibility helps in maintaining a sustainable approach rather than a rigid regimen that feels burdensome.

While designing this schedule, remember the importance of hydration. Water plays a critical role, not just in digestion and skin health, but in overall cellular function—something increasingly crucial during menopause. Ensuring you drink adequate water throughout your eating window not only aids in digestion and absorption of nutrients but also helps manage appetite and improve energy levels.

Developing and adhering to a structured eating schedule is your daily roadmap to navigating menopause with greater ease. By consistently aligning your meal timing, portions, and content with your body's needs, you empower yourself to manage this transitional phase with vigor, resilience, and tranquility. Each meal, each snack, timed and selected carefully, contributes significantly to this transformative phase of life, supporting you in embracing menopause not as a struggle, but as a passage to rediscover your body and its needs.

Essential Shopping List for Smart Buyers

As you venture into creating meals that support your journey through menopause, the cornerstone of your success is rooted in what you choose at the grocery store. Your food shopping habits set the stage for your dietary overhaul, ensuring that every meal reflects your commitment to manage weight, balance hormones, and enhance your overall wellness. Let's envision transforming your shopping list into a powerful tool for healthy living, filled with items that promise to nourish and rejuvenate your body.

When you enter the grocery store, view each aisle as an opportunity to make choices that align with your health goals. Begin with the perimeter of the store—often home to fresh produce, dairy, and proteins—which are essential for an anti-inflammatory and hormone-balancing diet. Picture yourself selecting vibrant vegetables and fruits, which are not just ingredients, but components packed with vitamins, minerals, and antioxidants, key in fighting inflammation and supporting cellular health.

Visualize reaching for leafy greens like spinach, kale, and Swiss chard. These aren't just sides for your dishes; they're nutrient powerhouses, rich in iron and calcium, which become increasingly important in your menopausal years. Pair these with colorful vegetables such as bell peppers, carrots, and beetroots, which add visual delight and a plethora of phytonutrients to your meals.

Next, think about your protein sources. Envision choosing wild-caught salmon, rich in omega-3 fatty acids, crucial for heart health and cognitive function, or lean poultry, which provides high-quality protein without the added fats that can exacerbate menopausal weight gain. When you select eggs, consider the enriched omega-3 options, which bolster your intake of those essential fats.

As you move towards the dairy section, imagine opting for high-protein, low-sugar options like Greek yogurt or kefir, which provide probiotics essential for gut health—an important aspect as gastrointestinal issues can often increase during menopause.

In the aisles, your focus shifts to whole grains and legumes. Picture yourself picking up quinoa, brown rice, or barley—whole grains that offer a hearty base for meals without spiking your blood sugar. Among legumes, visualize lentils or chickpeas, versatile and fiber-rich, supporting digestion and providing steady energy.

Your cart is not complete without healthy fats. Reach for avocados, nuts like almonds and walnuts, and seeds such as flaxseed or chia seeds. These are not mere add-ons but are crucial for their anti-inflammatory properties and their ability to support hormonal balance.

While spices and herbs might seem minor, picture these as powerful tools in your culinary arsenal. Turmeric, for instance, is not just a spice; it's a potent anti-inflammatory agent. Similarly, cinnamon can help regulate your blood sugar levels, and herbs like sage and basil add flavor without calories, encouraging you to enjoy your food while sticking to your health goals.

As you round out your shopping, consider the role of beverages. Envision replacing high-sugar drinks with green tea or herbal teas like chamomile, which not only hydrate but also provide compounds that aid in reducing menopause symptoms such as hot flashes and night sweats.

This shopping list, when transformed into a weekly habit, acts as a blueprint for your nutrient intake, a reflection of your dedication to your health through and beyond menopause. Each item on your list carries a purpose, each selection a step toward a healthier, more vibrant you.

Approach this weekly ritual with the enthusiasm of an artist selecting their palette. The grocery store is your studio, and your cart is the canvas. Each item you choose contributes to the masterpiece of your health. With each visit, you become more adept at identifying the foods that best support your journey, tailoring your selections to fit your evolving nutritional needs.

Moreover, shopping with this level of intention does more than just fill your pantry; it empowers you. It shifts your mindset from passive consumer to active health advocate. You are not merely shopping; you are curating a collection of ingredients that will form the basis of meals designed to enhance your life during menopause.

Incorporate this purposeful approach in your shopping routine, and watch how it transforms not just your diet, but your approach to health during menopause. Each meal planned with these carefully chosen ingredients will serve as a testament to your commitment to nurturing your body through one of its most transformative phases.

Preparing Your Kitchen for Dietary Success

Embracing the Galveston Diet during menopause means preparing not just your mind and body but also your kitchen—a crucial environment that can significantly influence your dietary success. As we delve into preparing your kitchen, envision this as an opportunity to create a sanctuary that supports your health goals, tailored to foster an inviting atmosphere that encourages nutritional abundance and ease of meal preparation.

First, consider the space's organization. The layout and organization of your kitchen can greatly affect how efficiently and enjoyably you prepare your meals. Picture opening your cabinets and finding exactly what you need without a second thought—this is the simplicity to strive for. Invest in organizational tools like clear containers that allow you to see your healthy grains, nuts, and seeds at a glance. Label everything distinctly, so choosing ingredients becomes an effortless task.

Your refrigerator is more than a cooling appliance; it's your garden of fresh produce and healthy substitutes. Organize it to prioritize accessibility to wholesome foods. Imagine placing pre-cut vegetables on middle shelves at eye level, making it the first thing you see when you open the door—a small yet potent reminder of your commitment every time you reach for a snack. Keep fruits in a visible basket to encourage natural sweet fixes instead of reaching for processed sugar options.

Freezers shouldn't be underestimated either. Often seen just as storage for leftovers, reimagine it as a resource for preserving the nutrient quality of seasonal produce and lean proteins bought in bulk. Store portions of fish, poultry, and even portions of antioxidant-rich berries in an organized manner to make meal preparation quicker and healthier choices easier.

The pantry is another pivotal aspect of your kitchen setup. Remove items that contradict your dietary goals and replace them with key staples of the Galveston Diet. Stock it with various spices that not only flavor your dishes but also offer health benefits, like turmeric for its anti-inflammatory properties and cinnamon for blood sugar regulation. Storing whole grains in clear, airtight containers not only keeps them fresh but also encourages you to use them.

Utensils and appliances play a supporting role in your kitchen's functionality. High-quality knives make chopping vegetables more enjoyable and less of a chore. A sturdy blender is essential for those morning smoothies packed with fibers and proteins. Consider tools like slow cookers or pressure cookers, which can help you prepare wholesome meals without the strain of constant monitoring, making your diet regimen more manageable and less time-consuming.

Lighting and ambiance are elements often overlooked in kitchen preparation. Adequate lighting is crucial—not just for safety and ease of cooking but also for the general appeal of your cooking space. Good lighting can elevate your mood and enhance your motivation to cook. Additionally, incorporate elements that make your kitchen inviting, like having a small radio for music or placing a few potted herbs on the windowsill, engaging your senses and enticing you to spend time preparing nourishing meals.

Hygiene and safety should be engrained habits. Ensure cutting boards are sanitized, and knives are sharpened; accidents and clutter only detract from your culinary experience. Regularly clean your oven, stovetop, and other appliances to maintain a healthy and inspiring environment that echoes cleanliness and order.

Emotionally connecting with your space is just as necessary. Personalize your kitchen with touches that reflect your style and make the space truly yours. Whether it's through artwork, color schemes, or decorative motifs, these personal touches can significantly boost your joy and satisfaction in utilizing this space.

Lastly, sustainability in your kitchen is not just a trend but a lifestyle choice that aligns with being mindful about your health and the environment. Incorporate practices such as composting or recycling, and consider using eco-friendly cleaning products. Not only do these habits make your kitchen an emblem of health, but they also contribute positively to the environment.

By optimizing your kitchen in these ways, you transform it from a mere room in your home to a powerhouse tailored to support your journey through menopause. This space becomes not just a place to cook, but a vital tool in your daily commitment to a healthier, more balanced lifestyle.

Tips for Weekly Meal Preparations

Imagine starting each week with a sense of calm and control, knowing that your meals are planned, prepared, and aligned with your health goals during menopause. Weekly meal preparation is not just a practical exercise; it's a ritual that sets the tone for a nourishing week ahead. This practice can be the cornerstone of successfully implementing the Galveston Diet, ensuring consistent, balanced, and beneficial meals throughout the week.

Embarking on this journey requires a blend of planning, flexibility, and creativity. Begin by setting aside a specific time each week, perhaps Sunday afternoon or Monday morning, to map out your meals. This isn't about rigidly planning every bite, but rather sketching a dietary blueprint that respects your body's needs and your lifestyle's demands.

Start with visualizing your week: Consider your schedule – which days might you be late home? When do you have more time to indulge in cooking? Some days will need quick-prep meals or slow cooker recipes that can simmer without supervision. Others might allow the luxury of experimenting with new recipes or techniques.

Drafting a meal plan should involve a careful balance of macronutrients—proteins, fats, and carbohydrates—ensuring they align with the Galveston Diet principles. Think of your plate as a canvas, where each mealtime adds color through vegetables, protein, and whole grains or legumes. Integrate variety to avoid dietary boredom — switch between poultry, fish, legumes, and lean cuts of meat across the week. Diversity in vegetables and fruits ensures a broad spectrum of nutrients which are essential during menopause for hormonal balance and mental health.

Once your meal plan is outlined, the next step is creating a shopping list that reflects your needs for the week. This practice avoids impulse purchases, keeps your budget in check, and ensures you have all the necessary ingredients for your planned meals, reducing mid-week store runs which can disrupt your dietary intentions.

The actual meal preparation begins by prepping ingredients in advance. Consider washing and chopping vegetables for ready-access snacking or quick assembly. Cooking grains or legumes in bulk can save significant time, allowing for easy side dishes or robust salad additions. Roasting a tray of mixed vegetables or preparing a large salad can provide nutritious options that are easily integrated into various meals.

Strategically use your kitchen tools and appliances to maximize efficiency. A food processor can quickly chop or shred items, slow cookers can develop deep flavors with minimal supervision, and pressure cookers reduce cooking time dramatically, which is a boon for preparing whole grains and legumes.

As you cook, remind yourself of the flexibility in your plan. If a particular dish is a hit, it might show up again in the week's plan as a new variation. Leftover grilled chicken can be repurposed into salads or wraps for lunch the following day, and a batch of quinoa cooked on Monday can find its way into different culinary creations throughout the week.

Furthermore, embracing the art of seasoning and marinating can transform the same ingredients into diverse, flavorful meals. Experiment with herbs and spices—like turmeric, ginger, or basil—which align with the anti-inflammatory focus of the Galveston Diet. They engage your senses, reduce monotony, and increase satisfaction with your meals, making the diet a pleasurable rather than strictly medicinal part of your life.

Effective meal preparation also involves mindful storage. Use clear, airtight containers to keep prepped components fresh and visible. Labeling items with dates ensures that you use them within their optimal freshness period, maintaining quality and taste.

Engage with others in your household during this process, making it interactive and enjoyable. This not only divides the labor but also increases commitment to healthy eating across your family. It turns meal preparation into a shared venture, reinforcing your dietary goals through collective effort.

Lastly, reflect on each week's meals. Which dishes were successful? What didn't work out as planned? This reflection is not about critique but learning and adapting your approach to continuously fine-tune your strategy. This ongoing process keeps the meal prep dynamic and responsive to your evolving dietary needs during menopause.

In sum, weekly meal preparation is your proactive step toward embracing a lifestyle that priorities nutritional richness and hormonal balance. It's about making thoughtful, informed food choices that sustain not just your body but also your spirit and joy in eating, ensuring longevity and health throughout your menopausal years.

6.Energizing Mornings: Breakfast Recipes

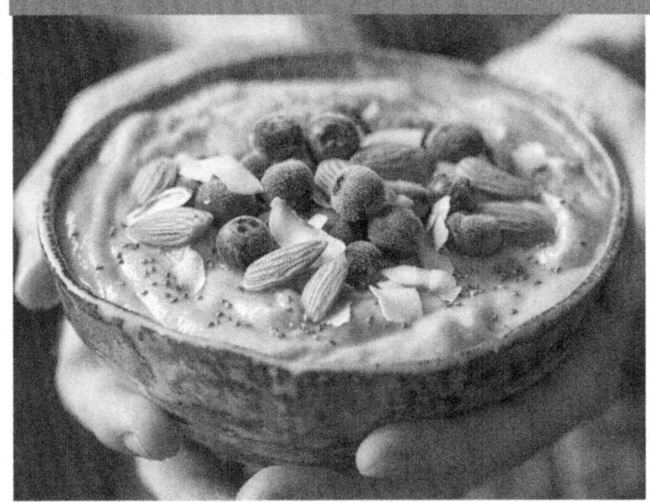

Mornings during menopause can sometimes feel like a slow ascent from a foggy bottom. As your body adapts to new rhythms, a nurturing start can set the tone for the entire day. Realizing the power of a nutrient-packed breakfast is pivotal, especially when your body is navigating the complex wave of hormonal adjustments that menopause presents.

Imagine stepping into your kitchen, greeted by the soft morning light. Here is where your day begins—a place of transformation and rejuvenation. In your hands, ingredients that do more than just satiate—they balance and heal. Every breakfast recipe has been crafted not only to meet your taste buds with delight but also to infuse your body with energy that lasts, stabilizes your hormones, and curtails the inflammation that can escalate during menopause.

Through the recipes in this chapter, we'll explore how smoothies and bowls can become a canvas for antioxidant-rich fruits, flaxseeds for omega-3s, and yogurt or almond milk for that creamy texture that keeps you full longer. We'll revel in the hearty, comforting embrace of proteins in forms that keep cooking simple yet exciting—whether it's a savory turkey sausage patty beside a sprig of rosemary or eggs scrambled softly with spinach and mushrooms.

Then, there are porridges—an age-old breakfast staple. But forget the mundane oatmeal; we're talking about quinoa porridge stirred gently with almond milk, topped with a swirl of agave and a handful of walnuts for a meal that supports blood sugar control.

The art of breakfast is not just in the preparation, but in its capacity to transform your health. Each recipe is a building block towards a resilient body that can embrace menopause with strength. These morning meals aren't just food; they are your first steps each day on the path to hormonal balance and well-being—a delicious promise of vitality and relief from the menopausal symptoms that challenge so many.

Let's warm our kitchens with these energizing recipes and light up our mornings with possibilities.

Smoothies and Bowls to Start the Day

Golden Turmeric Smoothie Bowl

Preparation Time: 10 min

Cooking Time: none

Mode of Cooking: Blending

Servings: 2 Serv.

Ingredients:

- 1 cup frozen mango chunks
- 1 ripe banana
- 1/2 cup coconut milk
- 1 tsp turmeric powder
- 1 Tbsp chia seeds
- 1 Tbsp honey
- 1 tsp freshly grated ginger
- 1/4 tsp cinnamon
- 1 Tbsp flaxseed meal
- 1/4 cup water

Directions:

1. Combine mango, banana, coconut milk, turmeric, chia seeds, honey, ginger, cinnamon, flaxseed meal, and water in a blender
2. Blend until smooth and creamy
3. Pour into two bowls and add toppings as desired

Tips:

- Use toppings like sliced almonds, coconut flakes, or blueberries for added texture and nutrients
- Incorporate a scoop of protein powder to enhance the smoothie's protein content if desired

Nutritional Values: Calories: 244, Fat: 7g, Carbs: 42g, Protein: 3g, Sugar: 29g, Sodium: 32mg, Potassium: 431mg, Cholesterol: 0mg

Spirulina Protein Bowl

Preparation Time: 8 min
Cooking Time: none
Mode of Cooking: Blending
Servings: 1
Ingredients:

- 1 ripe avocado
- 1 tsp spirulina powder
- 1 cup spinach leaves
- ½ cup Greek yogurt, unsweetened
- 1 Tbsp pumpkin seeds
- 1 Tbsp hemp seeds
- ½ green apple, chopped
- 1 cup almond milk
- ½ tsp vanilla extract
- 1 Tbsp lemon juice

Directions:

1. Pour almond milk, spinach, apple, avocado, spirulina powder, and lemon juice into a blender
2. Blend until smooth
3. Add Greek yogurt and blend briefly to incorporate
4. Pour into a bowl and sprinkle with pumpkin seeds and hemp seeds

Tips:

- Add a drizzle of agave syrup if a sweeter taste is preferred
- Consider sprinkling ground flaxseed on top for an extra fiber boost

Nutritional Values: Calories: 321, Fat: 21g, Carbs: 22g, Protein: 12g, Sugar: 9g, Sodium: 178mg, Potassium: 659mg, Cholesterol: 5mg

Acai Antioxidant Awakening Bowl

Preparation Time: 15 min
Cooking Time: none
Mode of Cooking: Blending
Servings: 2
Ingredients:

- 2 frozen acai berry packets
- 1 banana
- ½ cup mixed berries (blueberries, strawberries)
- 1 cup spinach leaves
- 1 Tbsp coconut oil
- 1 Tbsp almond butter
- 1 tsp ground flaxseeds
- ½ cup almond milk
- 1 tsp honey

Directions:

1. Blend acai packets, banana, mixed berries, spinach, and almond milk until smooth
2. Add coconut oil, almond butter, flaxseeds, and honey to the mixture and blend until perfectly smooth
3. Divide the blend into bowls and garnish with your choice of seeds and fruits

Tips:

- Sprinkle some bee pollen on top for an immune system boost
- For a crunchier texture, add granola on top before serving

Nutritional Values: Calories: 267, Fat: 14g, Carbs: 32g, Protein: 4g, Sugar: 17g, Sodium: 41mg, Potassium: 449mg, Cholesterol: 0mg

Cocoa & Beet Detox Smoothie Bowl

Preparation Time: 12 min
Cooking Time: none
Mode of Cooking: Blending
Servings: 1
Ingredients:

- 1 medium beet, cooked and sliced
- 1 ripe banana
- 2 Tbsp raw cocoa powder
- 1 Tbsp almond butter
- ½ cup Greek yogurt
- 1 Tbsp honey
- ½ tsp ground cinnamon
- 1 cup water

Directions:

1. Blend beet, banana, cocoa powder, almond butter, Greek yogurt, honey, cinnamon, and water until smooth
2. Taste and adjust sweetness if necessary with additional honey

3. Serve in a bowl and top with sliced banana and a sprinkle of chia seeds

Tips:

- For added protein, mix in a scoop of your favorite protein powder
- Top with almonds or walnuts for healthy fats and extra crunch

Nutritional Values: Calories: 330, Fat: 12g, Carbs: 48g, Protein: 10g, Sugar: 32g, Sodium: 62mg, Potassium: 702mg, Cholesterol: 3mg

Matcha Green Goddess Smoothie Bowl

Preparation Time: 10 min
Cooking Time: none
Mode of Cooking: Blending
Servings: 2
Ingredients:

- 1 tsp matcha green tea powder
- 1 ripe avocado
- 1 cup kale leaves
- ½ ripe banana
- 1 Tbsp chia seeds
- 2 dates, pitted
- ½ cup Greek yogurt
- 1 cup coconut water
- 1 Tbsp lemon juice

Directions:

1. Combine all ingredients in a blender and blend until smooth and evenly mixed
2. Pour into bowls and garnish with sliced kiwi, coconut flakes, and a sprinkle of bee pollen

Tips:

- Consider adding a scoop of vanilla protein powder for extra protein
- Use frozen banana to make the smoothie thicker and cooler

Nutritional Values: Calories: 219, Fat: 11g, Carbs: 26g, Protein: 7g, Sugar: 15g, Sodium: 78mg, Potassium: 548mg, Cholesterol: 4mg

Matcha Energy Bowl

Preparation Time: 12 min
Cooking Time: none
Mode of Cooking: Blending
Servings: 2
Ingredients:

- 2 C. fresh baby spinach
- 1 ripe avocado, pitted and scooped
- 1 tsp matcha powder
- 1 banana, sliced and frozen
- ½ C. Greek yogurt, unsweetened
- 1 C. almond milk
- 1 Tbsp honey
- 1 tsp spirulina powder
- Toppings: Sliced kiwi, pumpkin seeds, and a sprinkle of bee pollen

Directions:

1. Blend spinach, avocado, matcha powder, banana, Greek yogurt, almond milk, honey, and spirulina until creamy and smooth
2. Transfer to bowls and add toppings of sliced kiwi, pumpkin seeds, and bee pollen

Tips:

- To boost the protein content, add a scoop of your preferred vanilla protein powder
- Store any remaining matcha powder in a cool, dark place to maintain its vibrant color and health benefits

Nutritional Values: Calories: 320, Fat: 15g, Carbs: 35g, Protein: 10g, Sugar: 20g, Sodium: 50 mg, Potassium: 750 mg, Cholesterol: 5 mg

Breakfasts Rich in Protein

Spinach and Feta Breakfast Scramble

Preparation Time: Prep Time: 5 min.
Cooking Time: 10 min.
Mode of Cooking: Sautéing
Servings: 2

Ingredients:

- 4 large eggs, whisked
- 1 cup fresh spinach, roughly chopped

- 1/4 cup feta cheese, crumbled
- 1 Tbsp olive oil
- 1/4 tsp black pepper
- 1/4 tsp turmeric
- 1/4 cup onions, finely diced
- 1 clove garlic, minced

Directions:

1. Heat olive oil in a skillet over medium heat
2. Add onions and garlic; sauté until translucent
3. Add spinach and cook until wilted
4. Pour eggs into skillet; sprinkle turmeric and pepper
5. Stir gently until the eggs begin to set but remain slightly runny
6. Sprinkle feta cheese over the eggs; continue cooking until eggs are fully set

Tips:

- Serve with a slice of whole-grain toast for added fiber
- Adding a dash of chili flakes can enhance flavor and boost metabolism

Nutritional Values: Calories: 280, Fat: 21g, Carbs: 4g, Protein: 18g, Sugar: 2g, Sodium: 420 mg, Potassium: 234 mg, Cholesterol: 372 mg

Salmon and Avocado Omelette

Preparation Time: Prep Time: 8 min.

Cooking Time: 10 min.

Mode of Cooking: Frying

Servings: 1

Ingredients:

- 2 large eggs
- 1/2 avocado, sliced
- 2 oz. smoked salmon
- 1 Tbsp chives, chopped
- 1 tsp olive oil
- 1/4 tsp ground pepper
- 1/8 tsp sea salt

Directions:

1. Beat the eggs with salt and pepper in a bowl
2. Heat olive oil in a non-stick frying pan over medium heat
3. Pour the eggs into the pan, swirling to evenly coat the surface
4. As the edges set, lay slices of avocado and smoked salmon over one half of the omelette
5. Sprinkle with chives
6. Fold the omelette over and cook until the eggs are fully set

Tips:

- Top with a dollop of Greek yogurt for extra creaminess and a protein boost
- Serve immediately for best texture and flavor

Nutritional Values: Calories: 290, Fat: 22g, Carbs: 6g, Protein: 18g, Sugar: 1g, Sodium: 560 mg, Potassium: 450 mg, Cholesterol: 370 mg

Turkey and Quinoa Breakfast Bowl

Preparation Time: Prep Time: 15 min.

Cooking Time: 20 min.

Mode of Cooking: Boiling and Sautéing

Servings: 2

Ingredients:

- 1/2 cup quinoa, rinsed
- 1 cup water
- 1 Tbsp olive oil
- 6 oz. ground turkey
- 1/2 cup kale, chopped
- 1/4 cup red bell pepper, diced
- 1 Tbsp parsley, chopped
- 1 tsp paprika
- Salt and pepper to taste

Directions:

1. Bring water to a boil in a saucepan; add quinoa and simmer covered for 15 min. or until all water is absorbed
2. Heat olive oil in a skillet over medium heat
3. Add ground turkey and cook until browned
4. Add bell pepper and kale; sauté until softened
5. Stir in cooked quinoa, paprika, salt, and pepper; cook for an additional 2 min.
6. Garnish with fresh parsley before serving

Tips:

- Incorporate a squeeze of lemon for a fresh, tangy finish
- Quinoa can be cooked in bulk and stored in the fridge for quick prep on busy mornings

Nutritional Values: Calories: 315, Fat: 13g, Carbs: 27g, Protein: 23g, Sugar: 2g, Sodium: 75 mg, Potassium: 470 mg, Cholesterol: 80 mg

Cottage Cheese Pancakes

Preparation Time: Prep Time: 10 min.

Cooking Time: 5 min.

Mode of Cooking: Griddling

Servings: 2

Ingredients:

- 1/2 cup cottage cheese
- 1/2 cup oats
- 2 large eggs
- 1 Tbsp honey
- 1/2 tsp vanilla extract
- 1/4 tsp cinnamon
- 1 Tbsp coconut oil for cooking

Directions:

1. Place cottage cheese, oats, eggs, honey, vanilla, and cinnamon in a blender; blend until smooth
2. Heat coconut oil over medium heat on a griddle
3. Pour batter to form pancakes, cook until bubbles form on the surface and edges are dry, then flip and finish cooking

Tips:

- Serve with fresh berries and a drizzle of raw honey for added antioxidants and sweetness
- These pancakes store well in the refrigerator for a quick reheat during busy mornings

Nutritional Values: Calories: 255, Fat: 10g, Carbs: 26g, Protein: 15g, Sugar: 8g, Sodium: 350 mg, Potassium: 180 mg, Cholesterol: 185 mg

Greek Yogurt Smoothie Bowl

Preparation Time: Prep Time: 10 min.

Cooking Time: none

Mode of Cooking: Blending

Servings: 1

Ingredients:

- 1 cup Greek yogurt
- 1/2 banana, sliced
- 1/4 cup frozen blueberries
- 2 Tbsp chia seeds
- 1 Tbsp almond butter
- 1 tsp honey
- 1/4 tsp ground flaxseed

Directions:

1. Combine Greek yogurt, banana, blueberries, almond butter, and honey in a blender; blend until smooth
2. Pour into a bowl and sprinkle with chia seeds and ground flaxseed

Tips:

- Top with a handful of granola for added texture and fiber
- Customize with a variety of fruits and seeds depending on preferences and seasonal availability

Nutritional Values: Calories: 365, Fat: 15g, Carbs: 38g, Protein: 22g, Sugar: 20g, Sodium: 65 mg, Potassium: 350 mg, Cholesterol: 10 mg

Savory Spinach and Feta Breakfast Muffins

Preparation Time: 15 min

Cooking Time: 25 min

Mode of Cooking: Baking

Servings: 12

Ingredients:

- 2 C. whole wheat flour
- 1 Tbsp baking powder
- 1/2 tsp salt
- 2 large eggs
- 1 C. Greek yogurt
- 1/4 C. olive oil
- 1 C. feta cheese, crumbled
- 1 C. spinach, finely chopped
- 1/4 C. sun-dried tomatoes, chopped
- 1/2 C. skim milk

Directions:

1. Preheat oven to 350°F (175°C)
2. Mix flour, baking powder, and salt in a bowl
3. In another bowl, whisk eggs, Greek yogurt, and oil
4. Combine wet and dry mixtures
5. Fold in feta, spinach, and sun-dried tomatoes
6. Gradually add milk to achieve a batter consistency
7. Spoon into muffin tins and bake for 25 min.

Tips:

- Use silicone muffin pans for easy release without greasing
- For a vegan version, substitute eggs with flaxseed eggs and dairy with plant-based alternatives

Nutritional Values: Calories: 180, Fat: 9g, Carbs: 18g, Protein: 8g, Sugar: 2g, Sodium: 210 mg, Potassium: 134 mg, Cholesterol: 55 mg

Cozy and Satisfying Porridge Options

Quinoa Apple Cinnamon Porridge

Preparation Time: 10 min
Cooking Time: 15 min
Mode of Cooking: Stovetop
Servings: 2
Ingredients:

- 1 C. quinoa, rinsed
- 2 C. almond milk
- 1 large apple, peeled and grated
- 1 tsp cinnamon
- 1 Tbsp honey
- 1/4 C. chopped walnuts
- Pinch of salt

Directions:

1. Combine quinoa, almond milk, and salt in a medium saucepan and bring to a boil
2. Reduce heat to low and simmer covered for 15 min until quinoa is cooked
3. Stir in grated apple, cinnamon, and honey and cook for an additional 2 min
4. Serve hot, garnished with chopped walnuts

Tips:

- Stir occasionally to prevent sticking and enhance texture
- Add a spoonful of flaxseeds for extra fiber and omega-3's
- Enjoy with a dollop of Greek yogurt to add protein

Nutritional Values: Calories: 295, Fat: 9g, Carbs: 47g, Protein: 8g, Sugar: 12g, Sodium: 30 mg, Potassium: 239 mg, Cholesterol: 0 mg

Savory Turmeric Steel-Cut Oats

Preparation Time: 5 min
Cooking Time: 25 min
Mode of Cooking: Stovetop
Servings: 4
Ingredients:

- 1 C. steel-cut oats
- 4 C. low-sodium vegetable broth
- 1 tsp turmeric powder
- 1/2 C. chopped carrots
- 1/2 C. diced red bell peppers
- 1/4 C. chopped green onions
- Salt to taste
- Black pepper to taste

Directions:

1. Bring vegetable broth to a boil in a saucepan
2. Add steel-cut oats and turmeric, reduce heat to a simmer
3. Cook uncovered for 20 min, stirring occasionally
4. In the last 5 min, add carrots, bell peppers, and green onions
5. Season with salt and pepper

Tips:

- Serve with a sprinkle of fresh parsley for enhanced flavor and color
- Can be topped with a poached egg for added protein

Nutritional Values: Calories: 178, Fat: 3g, Carbs: 30g, Protein: 7g, Sugar: 2g, Sodium: 58 mg, Potassium: 221 mg, Cholesterol: 0 mg

Buckwheat and Chia Porridge

Preparation Time: 8 min
Cooking Time: 20 min
Mode of Cooking: Stovetop
Servings: 3
Ingredients:

- 1/2 C. buckwheat groats
- 1/4 C. chia seeds
- 2.5 C. coconut milk
- 1 tsp vanilla extract
- 1 Tbsp maple syrup

- Pinch of salt

Directions:

1. Combine buckwheat groats, chia seeds, coconut milk, and salt in a saucepan and soak for 8 min
2. Bring to a boil, then reduce heat to low and simmer for 20 min
3. Remove from heat and stir in vanilla extract and maple syrup

Tips:

- Let it sit for a few minutes to thicken before serving
- Serve with a handful of fresh berries for extra antioxidants
- Add a touch of cinnamon for a warming effect

Nutritional Values: Calories: 336, Fat: 19g, Carbs: 34g, Protein: 8g, Sugar: 7g, Sodium: 29 mg, Potassium: 177 mg, Cholesterol: 0 mg

Spiced Pumpkin Millet Porridge

Preparation Time: 10 min
Cooking Time: 30 min
Mode of Cooking: Stovetop
Servings: 2
Ingredients:

- 1/2 C. millet, rinsed
- 2 C. water
- 1/2 C. pumpkin puree
- 1 tsp pumpkin pie spice
- 1 Tbsp almond butter
- 1 Tbsp molasses
- 1/4 tsp salt

Directions:

1. Toast millet in a dry skillet over medium heat until fragrant, about 3 min
2. Add water and salt, bring to a boil, then cover and simmer for 25 min
3. Stir in pumpkin puree, pumpkin pie spice, almond butter, and molasses, cook for an additional 5 min

Tips:

- Top with a sprinkle of toasted pumpkin seeds for crunch and protein
- Serve with a splash of almond milk for creaminess

Nutritional Values: Calories: 308, Fat: 8g, Carbs: 53g, Protein: 6g, Sugar: 8g, Sodium: 350 mg, Potassium: 262 mg, Cholesterol: 0 mg

Matcha Green Tea Oatmeal

Preparation Time: 5 min
Cooking Time: 10 min
Mode of Cooking: Stovetop
Servings: 2
Ingredients:

- 1 C. rolled oats
- 2 C. water or milk of choice
- 1 tsp matcha green tea powder
- 1 Tbsp honey
- 1/2 tsp vanilla extract
- Pinch of salt

Directions:

1. Bring water or milk to a boil in a saucepan
2. Add oats and salt, reduce heat, and simmer for 10 min, stirring occasionally
3. Remove from heat and stir in matcha powder, honey, and vanilla extract

Tips:

- Serve with a topping of fresh kiwi or mango for a vibrant start to your day
- Consider adding a sprinkle of hemp seeds for added texture and protein

Nutritional Values: Calories: 237, Fat: 3g, Carbs: 42g, Protein: 6g, Sugar: 12g, Sodium: 24 mg, Potassium: 126 mg, Cholesterol: 0 mg

Golden Turmeric Millet Porridge

Preparation Time: 10 min.
Cooking Time: 20 min.
Mode of Cooking: Stovetop
Servings: 2
Ingredients:

- 1 cup millet, rinsed
- 3 cups water
- 1 tsp ground turmeric
- 1 Tbsp coconut oil
- 1 Tbsp honey
- ¼ tsp ground cinnamon
- A pinch of salt
- 2 Tbsp slivered almonds
- ½ cup diced mango

Directions:

1. Toast millet in a dry skillet over medium heat until lightly golden, stirring often
2. Add water, turmeric, coconut oil, honey, cinnamon, and salt to the skillet and bring to a boil
3. Reduce heat to low, cover, and simmer for 18 min. or until millet is tender and creamy
4. Serve hot topped with slivered almonds and diced mango

Tips:

- Add a dollop of Greek yogurt for added creaminess and protein
- Experiment with other fruits like blueberries or chopped apples for variety in flavor and texture

Nutritional Values: Calories: 308, Fat: 8g, Carbs: 55g, Protein: 6g, Sugar: 9g, Sodium: 120 mg, Potassium: 105 mg, Cholesterol: 0 mg

7.Nutrient-Rich Light Meals: Salads and Vegetables

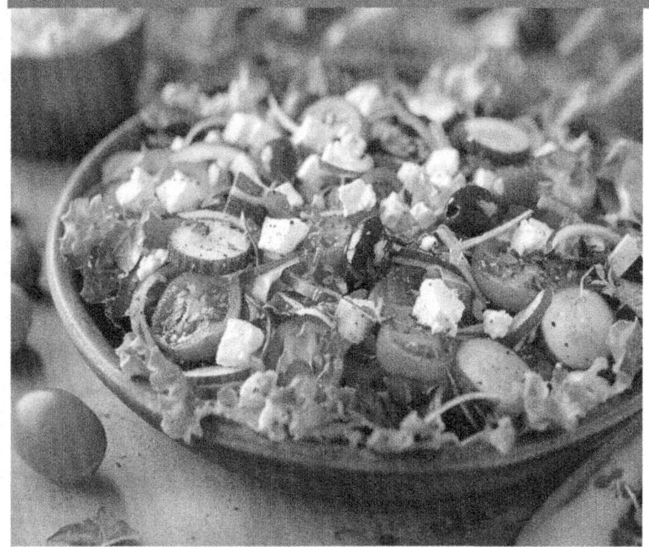

Imagine a garden where the colors vividly dance across your vision, where the crisp, fresh scents of various greens mingle with the sweet, intoxicating aroma of ripe vegetables. This isn't just any garden; it's the vibrant tableau from which our Nutrient-Rich Light Meals chapter draws its inspiration, focusing on salads and vegetables that combine both health and flavor in each bite.

For many women navigating the often turbulent waters of menopause, maintaining a diet that's both enriching and satisfying can seem like a daunting task. Yet, herein lies the beauty of integrating a rainbow of vegetables and inventive salads into your daily regimen. These dishes are not merely meals; they represent a potent lever in managing your weight, bolstering your health, and enhancing your energy levels—crucial elements during these transformative years.

Salads, often underrated, are a powerhouse of nutrients, fibers, and antioxidants. They can be a canvas for culinary creativity, integrating anti-inflammatory ingredients like leafy greens, nuts, and seeds, all of which are pivotal in balancing hormones and reducing menopause-related symptoms. Moreover, vegetables—whether raw, roasted, or steamed—bring comfort and variety to our plates, ensuring that each meal is a celebration of flavors and textures, enticing even to those in your family not bound by menopausal diet considerations.

In this chapter, the intention is to guide you away from the mundane salad stereotypes and introduce methods to elevate these dishes into something extraordinary. Here, you'll discover how to transform simple ingredients into nourishing creations that appeal to the palate and feed the body's needs during a period of life when nutrition is more critical than ever.

Embrace this journey through a garden of vibrancy and vitality. Let each recipe not only nourish your body but also rekindle a love for wholesome eating, hand-in-hand with the shifting tides of your body's needs.

Fresh and Flavorful Salad Creations

Mediterranean Crunch Salad

Preparation Time: 15 min
Cooking Time: none
Mode of Cooking: No Cooking
Servings: 4
Ingredients:

- 4 cups mixed salad greens
- 1/2 cup thin-sliced radicchio
- 1 red bell pepper, julienned
- 1 cucumber, deseeded and thin-sliced
- 1/4 cup thinly sliced red onion
- 10 cherry tomatoes, halved
- 1/4 cup kalamata olives, pitted and halved
- 1/4 cup crumbled feta cheese
- 2 Tbsp extra virgin olive oil
- 1 Tbsp red wine vinegar
- 1/2 tsp dried oregano
- Salt and pepper to taste

Directions:

1. Combine greens, radicchio, bell pepper, cucumber, onion, tomatoes, and olives in a large salad bowl
2. Whisk together olive oil, red wine vinegar, oregano, salt, and pepper in a small bowl
3. Pour dressing over salad and toss gently to coat
4. Sprinkle feta cheese on top before serving

Tips:

- Serve immediately for optimal freshness and crunch
- Pair with grilled fish or chicken for a balanced meal

Nutritional Values: Calories: 180, Fat: 15g, Carbs: 10g, Protein: 4g, Sugar: 4g, Sodium: 320 mg, Potassium: 250 mg, Cholesterol: 15 mg

Asian Sesame Edamame Salad

Preparation Time: 20 min
Cooking Time: none
Mode of Cooking: No Cooking
Servings: 4
Ingredients:

- 3 cups shelled edamame, cooked and cooled
- 1 cup shredded carrot
- 1 red bell pepper, thinly sliced
- 1/2 cup thinly sliced scallions
- 1/4 cup cilantro leaves
- 3 Tbsp sesame seeds, toasted
- 2 Tbsp sesame oil
- 2 Tbsp soy sauce
- 1 Tbsp rice vinegar
- 1 Tbsp honey
- 1 tsp grated ginger
- 1 garlic clove, minced

Directions:

1. Combine edamame, carrot, bell pepper, scallions, and cilantro in a salad bowl
2. In another bowl, combine sesame seeds, sesame oil, soy sauce, rice vinegar, honey, ginger, and garlic to make the dressing
3. Pour dressing over the salad and toss thoroughly
4. Chill before serving to blend the flavors

Tips:

- Garnish with extra sesame seeds for a textural contrast
- Adjust the sweetness with more or less honey according to taste

Nutritional Values: Calories: 220, Fat: 14g, Carbs: 17g, Protein: 12g, Sugar: 6g, Sodium: 430 mg, Potassium: 500 mg, Cholesterol: 0 mg

Roasted Beet and Citrus Salad

Preparation Time: 45 min
Cooking Time: 30 min
Mode of Cooking: Roasting
Servings: 4
Ingredients:

- 4 medium beets, trimmed, washed, and cubed
- 2 oranges, peeled and segments removed
- 1 grapefruit, peeled and segments removed
- 6 cups baby arugula
- 1/2 cup walnut halves, toasted
- 1/4 cup crumbled goat cheese
- 3 Tbsp extra virgin olive oil
- 2 Tbsp balsamic vinegar
- 1 tsp honey
- Salt and black pepper to taste

Directions:

1. Preheat oven to 400°F (204°C)
2. Roast beets on a lined baking sheet until tender, about 30 min
3. Allow beets to cool
4. In a large bowl, arrange arugula, then top with roasted beets, orange and grapefruit segments
5. Sprinkle walnuts and goat cheese over the top
6. Whisk together olive oil, balsamic vinegar, honey, salt, and pepper for the dressing
7. Drizzle dressing over the salad

Tips:

- Add a sprinkle of flax seeds for an extra nutritious boost
- Serving chilled enhances the flavors

Nutritional Values: Calories: 290, Fat: 20g, Carbs: 22g, Protein: 8g, Sugar: 15g, Sodium: 220 mg, Potassium: 540 mg, Cholesterol: 15 mg

Avocado and Quinoa Power Salad

Preparation Time: 15 min
Cooking Time: 15 min
Mode of Cooking: Boiling
Servings: 4
Ingredients:

- 1 cup quinoa, rinsed
- 2 cups water
- 1 ripe avocado, diced

- 1 cup cherry tomatoes, halved
- 1/2 cup corn kernels, cooked
- 1/2 cup black beans, rinsed and drained
- 1/4 cup chopped fresh cilantro
- 1 lime, juiced
- 2 Tbsp extra virgin olive oil
- Salt and pepper to taste

Directions:

1. Boil quinoa in water until fluffy and fully cooked, about 15 min; allow to cool
2. In a large bowl, combine cooled quinoa, avocado, tomatoes, corn, and black beans
3. Add cilantro, lime juice, and olive oil to the bowl
4. Season with salt and pepper
5. Toss all ingredients until well mixed

Tips:

- Serve as a stand-alone meal or as a side to lean proteins
- The lime juice prevents the avocado from browning if not serving immediately

Nutritional Values: Calories: 280, Fat: 15g, Carbs: 30g, Protein: 8g, Sugar: 3g, Sodium: 15 mg, Potassium: 680 mg, Cholesterol: 0 mg

Spicy Kale and Chickpea Toss

Preparation Time: 10 min
Cooking Time: none
Mode of Cooking: No Cooking
Servings: 4
Ingredients:

- 6 cups kale, stemmed and chopped
- 1 can (15 oz.) chickpeas, rinsed and drained
- 1/2 cup diced red onion
- 1/2 cup shredded carrot
- 1/4 cup pumpkin seeds
- 1/4 cup golden raisins
- 2 Tbsp olive oil
- 2 Tbsp apple cider vinegar
- 1 Tbsp sriracha sauce
- 1 tsp honey
- Salt and pepper to taste

Directions:

1. In a large serving bowl, combine kale, chickpeas, onion, carrot, pumpkin seeds, and raisins
2. In a small bowl, whisk together olive oil, vinegar, sriracha, honey, salt, and pepper to create the dressing
3. Pour dressing over the kale mixture and toss to coat thoroughly
4. Let sit for 5 min before serving to soften the kale

Tips:

- Massage the kale leaves with olive oil before adding other ingredients to tenderize them
- Adjust the level of spiciness by increasing or decreasing the sriracha sauce

Nutritional Values: Calories: 230, Fat: 10g, Carbs: 30g, Protein: 8g, Sugar: 10g, Sodium: 300 mg, Potassium: 450 mg, Cholesterol: 0 mg

Spicy Kale and Quinoa Black Bean Salad

Preparation Time: 20 min
Cooking Time: none
Mode of Cooking: No Cooking
Servings: 4
Ingredients:

- 1 cup quinoa, rinsed
- 2 cups water
- 4 cups kale, stems removed and leaves finely chopped
- 1 can black beans, drained and rinsed
- 1 red bell pepper, diced
- 1/4 cup red onion, finely chopped
- 1/4 cup cilantro, chopped
- 1 avocado, diced
- 1 lime, juiced
- 2 Tbsp olive oil
- 1 tsp smoked paprika
- 1/2 tsp cumin
- Salt and black pepper to taste

Directions:

1. Combine quinoa and water in a pot, bring to a boil, then cover and simmer for 15 min until water is absorbed
2. Fluff quinoa with a fork and allow to cool

3. In a large bowl, combine cooled quinoa, kale, black beans, bell pepper, onion, and cilantro
4. In a small bowl, whisk together lime juice, olive oil, smoked paprika, cumin, salt, and black pepper to make the dressing
5. Pour dressing over salad and mix thoroughly
6. Gently fold in diced avocado just before serving

Tips:

- Serve immediately or let sit in the refrigerator for flavors to meld
- Use a vegetable peeler to create thin slices of avocado for garnishing if desired
- Add a protein such as grilled chicken or tofu to make it a complete meal

Nutritional Values: Calories: 310, Fat: 14g, Carbs: 42g, Protein: 9g, Sugar: 4g, Sodium: 30mg, Potassium: 1017mg, Cholesterol: 0mg

Various Ways to Enjoy Vegetables: Roasted, Steamed, and Raw

Zesty Turmeric Roasted Cauliflower

Preparation Time: 10 min
Cooking Time: 25 min
Mode of Cooking: Roasting
Servings: 4
Ingredients:

- 1 large head cauliflower, cut into florets
- 2 Tbsp extra virgin olive oil
- 1 tsp turmeric
- 1/2 tsp garlic powder
- 1/4 tsp cayenne pepper
- Salt and black pepper to taste

Directions:

1. Preheat oven to 425°F (220°C)
2. In a large bowl, toss cauliflower florets with olive oil, turmeric, garlic powder, cayenne pepper, salt, and black pepper until evenly coated
3. Spread onto a baking sheet in a single layer and roast in the oven until golden and tender, about 25 min

Tips:

- Stir halfway through roasting to ensure even cooking
- Serve with a sprinkle of fresh parsley for added freshness and color

Nutritional Values: Calories: 107, Fat: 7g, Carbs: 10g, Protein: 3g, Sugar: 3g, Sodium: 30 mg, Potassium: 320 mg, Cholesterol: 0 mg

Garlic Lemon Steamed Asparagus

Preparation Time: 5 min
Cooking Time: 7 min
Mode of Cooking: Steaming
Servings: 4
Ingredients:

- 1 lb. asparagus, trimmed
- 1 Tbsp olive oil
- 2 cloves garlic, minced
- Juice of 1 lemon
- Salt and black pepper to taste

Directions:

1. Bring water to a boil in a pot fitted with a steamer basket
2. Place asparagus in the basket, cover, and steam until tender yet firm, about 7 min
3. In a small bowl, mix olive oil, minced garlic, lemon juice, salt, and black pepper
4. Drizzle over cooked asparagus before serving

Tips:

- For best flavor, serve immediately after dressing
- Lemon zest can be added for an extra zing
- Avoid overcooking to maintain crispness

Nutritional Values: Calories: 60, Fat: 3.6g, Carbs: 4g, Protein: 3g, Sugar: 2g, Sodium: 3 mg, Potassium: 230 mg, Cholesterol: 0 mg

Spicy Raw Carrot Ribbon Salad

Preparation Time: 15 min
Cooking Time: none
Mode of Cooking: No Cooking
Servings: 4
Ingredients:

- 5 large carrots, peeled and sliced into ribbons using a vegetable peeler
- 1/4 cup fresh cilantro, chopped
- 2 Tbsp toasted sesame oil
- 1 Tbsp apple cider vinegar
- 1 Tbsp honey
- 1 tsp sriracha sauce
- Salt and black pepper to taste

Directions:

1. In a large bowl, combine carrot ribbons and chopped cilantro
2. In a small bowl, whisk together sesame oil, apple cider vinegar, honey, sriracha sauce, salt, and black pepper
3. Pour dressing over the carrot mixture and toss to coat thoroughly

Tips:

- Allow sitting for 10 min for flavors to meld
- Add toasted sesame seeds for a nutty flavor and crunch
- Adjust the amount of sriracha based on your heat preference

Nutritional Values: Calories: 123, Fat: 7g, Carbs: 14g, Protein: 1g, Sugar: 10g, Sodium: 180 mg, Potassium: 360 mg, Cholesterol: 0 mg

Herb-Infused Mushroom and Pea Pod Stir-Fry

Preparation Time: 10 min
Cooking Time: 8 min
Mode of Cooking: Stir-Frying
Servings: 4
Ingredients:

- 2 cups mushrooms, sliced
- 1 cup pea pods
- 1 Tbsp olive oil
- 1 garlic clove, minced
- 1 Tbsp soy sauce (low sodium)
- 1 tsp fresh ginger, grated
- 1/4 cup fresh basil leaves, chopped
- 1/4 cup fresh mint leaves, chopped

Directions:

1. Heat olive oil in a large skillet over medium-high heat
2. Add garlic and ginger, sauté for 1 min
3. Add mushrooms and pea pods, stir-fry for about 7 min
4. Stir in soy sauce, basil, and mint, cook for an additional 1 min

Tips:

- Serve hot for best flavor
- Pair with a protein source like grilled chicken for a balanced meal
- Can be garnished with red pepper flakes for extra heat

Nutritional Values: Calories: 95, Fat: 7g, Carbs: 7g, Protein: 3g, Sugar: 3g, Sodium: 620 mg, Potassium: 295 mg, Cholesterol: 0 mg

Balsamic Glazed Beetroot Wedges

Preparation Time: 15 min
Cooking Time: 40 min
Mode of Cooking: Roasting
Servings: 4
Ingredients:

- 4 medium beetroots, cut into wedges
- 2 Tbsp balsamic vinegar
- 1 Tbsp olive oil
- 1 tsp thyme, dried
- Salt and black pepper to taste

Directions:

1. Preheat oven to 400°F (200°C)
2. In a bowl, toss beetroot wedges with olive oil, thyme, salt, and black pepper
3. Spread on a baking sheet and roast until tender, about 40 min, turning halfway through
4. Drizzle balsamic vinegar over roasted beetroots in the last 10 min of cooking

Tips:

- Allow to cool slightly before serving to enhance flavor absorption
- Serve alongside a green salad or as a side to lean protein

Nutritional Values: Calories: 58, Fat: 3.5g, Carbs: 6g, Protein: 1g, Sugar: 5g, Sodium: 65 mg, Potassium: 267 mg, Cholesterol: 0 mg

Charred Broccoli and Carrot Medley

Preparation Time: 10 min

Cooking Time: 15 min

Mode of Cooking: Roasting

Servings: 4

Ingredients:

- 1 lb broccoli, cut into florets
- ½ lb carrots, julienned
- 2 Tbsp olive oil
- 1 tsp garlic powder
- ½ tsp chili flakes
- Salt and pepper to taste
- 1 Tbsp lemon zest

Directions:

1. Preheat oven to 425°F (220°C)
2. Toss broccoli and carrots with olive oil, garlic powder, chili flakes, salt, and pepper
3. Spread on a baking sheet in a single layer
4. Roast for 15 min or until edges are crispy and tender
5. Sprinkle with lemon zest before serving

Tips:

- Serve with a drizzle of balsamic reduction for extra flavor
- Pair with grilled salmon or chicken for a balanced meal

Nutritional Values: Calories: 120, Fat: 7g, Carbs: 13g, Protein: 4g, Sugar: 4g, Sodium: 45 mg, Potassium: 470 mg, Cholesterol: 0 mg

Homemade Dressings and Dips

Turmeric Tahini Drizzle

Preparation Time: 10 min

Cooking Time: none

Mode of Cooking: No Cooking

Servings: 4

Ingredients:

- 3 Tbsp tahini
- 1 Tbsp extra virgin olive oil
- 1 Tbsp lemon juice
- 1 tsp ground turmeric
- 1/2 tsp garlic powder
- 1/4 tsp cayenne pepper
- Salt to taste
- Water as needed for consistency

Directions:

1. Combine tahini, olive oil, lemon juice, turmeric, garlic powder, cayenne pepper, and salt in a bowl
2. Whisk until smooth, adding water slowly until desired consistency is reached

Tips:

- Use as a dressing over roasted vegetables or as a dip for fresh cut veggies
- Store in an airtight container in the refrigerator for up to 5 days

Nutritional Values: Calories: 91, Fat: 8g, Carbs: 3g, Protein: 2g, Sugar: 0.4g, Sodium: 23 mg, Potassium: 44 mg, Cholesterol: 0 mg

Avocado Cilantro Lime Dressing

Preparation Time: 10 min

Cooking Time: none

Mode of Cooking: No Cooking

Servings: 4

Ingredients:

- 1 ripe avocado
- 1/4 cup fresh cilantro, chopped
- 1/4 cup lime juice
- 1/4 cup Greek yogurt
- 1 clove garlic, minced
- Salt and pepper to taste
- Water for thinning

Directions:

1. Scoop the avocado into a blender
2. Add cilantro, lime juice, Greek yogurt, and garlic
3. Blend until smooth, adding water as needed to achieve a pourable consistency

Tips:

- Drizzle over a mixed bean salad or use as a creamy dip for pita chips

- Can be refrigerated for up to 3 days in an airtight container

Nutritional Values: Calories: 80, Fat: 7g, Carbs: 4g, Protein: 1g, Sugar: 1g, Sodium: 30 mg, Potassium: 187 mg, Cholesterol: 1 mg

Ginger Sesame Vinaigrette

Preparation Time: 10 min
Cooking Time: none
Mode of Cooking: No Cooking
Servings: 4
Ingredients:

- 1/4 cup sesame oil
- 2 Tbsp rice vinegar
- 1 Tbsp soy sauce
- 1 Tbsp honey
- 1 tsp grated fresh ginger
- 1/2 tsp minced garlic
- 1 tsp sesame seeds
- Salt and pepper to taste

Directions:

1. Mix sesame oil, rice vinegar, soy sauce, honey, ginger, garlic, and sesame seeds in a small mixing bowl
2. Stir until well blended and season with salt and pepper to taste

Tips:

- Perfectly pairs with Asian-style salad or as a marinade for grilled chicken
- Keep refrigerated and use within 4 days for best freshness

Nutritional Values: Calories: 130, Fat: 12g, Carbs: 5g, Protein: 1g, Sugar: 4g, Sodium: 330 mg, Potassium: 0 mg, Cholesterol: 0 mg

Roasted Red Pepper and Walnut Pesto

Preparation Time: 15 min
Cooking Time: none
Mode of Cooking: No Cooking
Servings: 4
Ingredients:

- 1 cup roasted red peppers, drained
- 1/2 cup walnuts, toasted
- 1/4 cup grated Parmesan cheese
- 1/4 cup basil leaves
- 2 Tbsp olive oil
- 1 clove garlic, minced
- Salt to taste

Directions:

1. Place all ingredients in a food processor
2. Pulse until smooth and well combined, scraping down sides as necessary

Tips:

- Serve as a spread for sandwiches or mix into cooked pasta
- Store in the refrigerator in an airtight container for up to a week

Nutritional Values: Calories: 170, Fat: 16g, Carbs: 5g, Protein: 4g, Sugar: 2g, Sodium: 190 mg, Potassium: 50 mg, Cholesterol: 4 mg

Creamy Dill and Mustard Sauce

Preparation Time: 10 min
Cooking Time: none
Mode of Cooking: No Cooking
Servings: 4
Ingredients:

- 1/2 cup Greek yogurt
- 2 Tbsp Dijon mustard
- 1/4 cup chopped fresh dill
- 1 Tbsp lemon juice
- 1 tsp honey
- Salt and black pepper to taste

Directions:

1. In a bowl, combine Greek yogurt, Dijon mustard, chopped dill, lemon juice, and honey
2. Mix thoroughly until smooth
3. Season with salt and black pepper according to taste

Tips:

- Ideal as a dressing for potato salad or as a dip for vegetables
- To thin the sauce, add a small amount of water or milk
- Refrigerate and use within 5 days

Nutritional Values: Calories: 35, Fat: 0.5g, Carbs: 5g, Protein: 3g, Sugar: 3g, Sodium: 150 mg, Potassium: 60 mg, Cholesterol: 2 mg

Turmeric Tahini Dressing

Preparation Time: 5 min
Cooking Time: none
Mode of Cooking: No Cooking
Servings: 8
Ingredients:

- 3 Tbsp tahini
- 1 Tbsp extra virgin olive oil
- 2 Tbsp lemon juice
- 1 tsp turmeric powder
- 1 clove garlic, minced
- ½ tsp freshly ground black pepper
- ½ tsp sea salt
- 3 Tbsp water, to thin

Directions:

1. Whisk together tahini, olive oil, lemon juice, turmeric powder, minced garlic, black pepper, and sea salt in a bowl until smooth
2. Gradually add water to reach desired consistency

Tips:

- Add a touch of honey or maple syrup if a sweeter dressing is preferred
- Can be stored in an airtight container in the refrigerator for up to a week
- To enhance anti-inflammatory benefits, pair with a salad rich in leafy greens

Nutritional Values: Calories: 55, Fat: 5g, Carbs: 2g, Protein: 1g, Sugar: 0g, Sodium: 150 mg, Potassium: 44 mg, Cholesterol: 0 mg

8.Aquatic Delights: Fish and Seafood Dishes

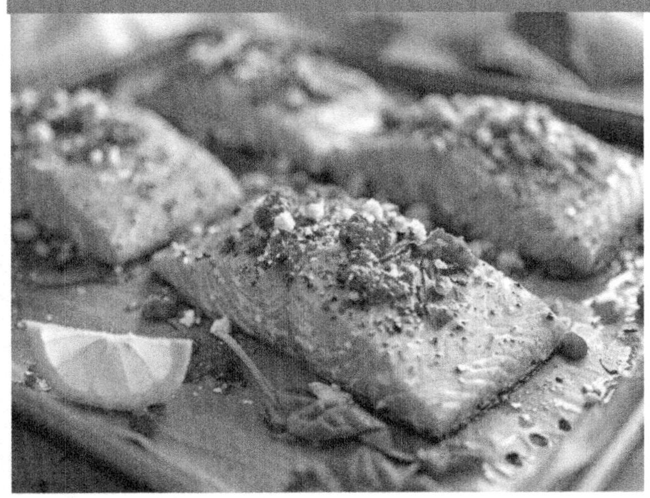

The allure of fish and seafood in our diets transcends mere taste; it is a profound embrace of nature's gift to our hormonal health, especially during menopause. As we explore the vibrant world of aquatic delights in this chapter, we're not just sharing recipes. We're diving into a sea of benefits that support hormonal balance and provide anti-inflammatory advantages, crucial during the challenging phase of menopause.

Imagine the gentle, rhythmic sound of ocean waves, a soothing reminder of the purity and freshness of seafood. Incorporating fish and seafood into our diets is akin to bringing the tranquility and nourishment of the sea directly to our dining tables. Each dish prepared is not just a meal but a celebration of life's natural rhythms, aligning our bodies and spirits with the healing pace of nature.

With fish and seafood, variety is as vast as the ocean itself. From the quick simplicity of seared scallops to the slow-cooked richness of a fish stew, these recipes are designed to enhance your metabolic health without sacrificing flavor. Rich in omega-3 fatty acids, seafood enhances our body's anti-inflammatory responses—so crucial in alleviating those persistent menopausal symptoms like hot flashes and mood swings.

It's important to consider sustainability and the environmental impact of our choices, selecting seafood that is not only beneficial to our health but also responsibly sourced. This mindfulness ensures that each dish brings to us the very best from the seas and rivers without depleting those precious natural reserves.

In this chapter, we do more than cook; we connect. Each recipe is an opportunity to nourish not only our bodies but also our connection with the environment and with one another. Whether it's a family gathering or a quiet meal alone, let these dishes be a potent reminder of the delicate, yet profound, influence of our dietary choices on our overall menopausal wellness. Enjoy the journey through each delightful, healthful recipe, and may every bite bring you closer to balance and vitality.

Methods for Grilling and Baking Fish

Mediterranean Stuffed Salmon

Preparation Time: 15 min

Cooking Time: 20 min

Mode of Cooking: Baking

Servings: 4

Ingredients:

- 4 salmon fillets, 6 oz each
- 2 Tbsp olive oil
- 1 cup fresh spinach, chopped
- ½ cup feta cheese, crumbled
- ¼ cup sun-dried tomatoes, chopped
- 2 cloves garlic, minced
- 1 lemon, zest and juice
- Salt and pepper to taste

Directions:

1. Preheat oven to 375°F (190°C)
2. In a skillet, heat 1 Tbsp olive oil and sauté garlic and spinach until wilted
3. Remove from heat and mix in feta cheese, sun-dried tomatoes, lemon zest, and juice
4. Cut a slit in each salmon fillet to create a pocket and stuff with the spinach mixture
5. Place on a baking sheet, drizzle with remaining olive oil, and season with salt and pepper
6. Bake for 20 min or until salmon is cooked through

Tips:

- Serve with a wedge of lemon for extra zest
- Pair with a side of quinoa for a complete meal

Nutritional Values: Calories: 297, Fat: 17g, Carbs: 6g, Protein: 29g, Sugar: 2g, Sodium: 160 mg, Potassium: 800 mg, Cholesterol: 75 mg

Citrus Herb Grilled Trout

Preparation Time: 10 min
Cooking Time: 8 min
Mode of Cooking: Grilling
Servings: 2
Ingredients:

- 2 whole trout, cleaned and scaled
- 1 orange, sliced
- 1 lemon, sliced
- 2 Tbsp fresh dill, chopped
- 2 Tbsp fresh parsley, chopped
- 4 Tbsp olive oil
- Salt and pepper to taste

Directions:

1. Preheat grill to medium-high or 375°F (190°C)
2. Rinse trout and pat dry
3. Stuff each trout with orange slices, lemon slices, dill, and parsley
4. Rub outside with olive oil and season with salt and pepper
5. Grill each side for 4 min or until the skin is crisp and the flesh is opaque

Tips:

- Grill on a cedar plank for an added smoky flavor
- Serve immediately for the best texture

Nutritional Values: Calories: 345, Fat: 21g, Carbs: 5g, Protein: 33g, Sugar: 2g, Sodium: 95 mg, Potassium: 560 mg, Cholesterol: 87 mg

Honey-Lime Baked Cod

Preparation Time: 10 min
Cooking Time: 15 min
Mode of Cooking: Baking
Servings: 4
Ingredients:

- 4 cod fillets, 6 oz each
- 2 Tbsp honey
- Juice of 2 limes
- 1 Tbsp soy sauce
- 1 tsp grated ginger
- 2 Tbsp olive oil
- Salt and pepper to taste

Directions:

1. Preheat oven to 400°F (204°C)
2. In a bowl, whisk together honey, lime juice, soy sauce, grated ginger, and olive oil
3. Place cod fillets in a baking dish and pour marinade over them
4. Season with salt and pepper
5. Bake for 15 min or until fish flakes easily

Tips:

- Baste the cod with the marinade halfway through cooking for extra flavor
- Serve with steamed broccoli and brown rice for a wholesome meal

Nutritional Values: Calories: 230, Fat: 7g, Carbs: 12g, Protein: 30g, Sugar: 9g, Sodium: 350 mg, Potassium: 740 mg, Cholesterol: 60 mg

Spicy Grilled Tilapia with Avocado Salsa

Preparation Time: 15 min
Cooking Time: 10 min
Mode of Cooking: Grilling
Servings: 4
Ingredients:

- 4 tilapia fillets, 6 oz each
- 2 tsp chili powder
- 1 tsp cumin
- 1 ripe avocado, diced
- 1 small red onion, diced
- 1 jalapeño, seeded and minced
- Juice of 1 lime
- 2 Tbsp cilantro, chopped
- 2 Tbsp olive oil
- Salt and pepper to taste

Directions:

1. Preheat grill to high or 400°F (204°C)
2. Mix chili powder and cumin, and rub onto tilapia fillets
3. In a bowl, combine avocado, red onion, jalapeño, lime juice, cilantro, and olive oil
4. Season salsa with salt and pepper

5. Grill tilapia for 5 min per side or until fully cooked
6. Serve topped with avocado salsa

Tips:

- Avoid overcooking the tilapia to maintain moisture
- Serve with a refreshing side of cucumber salad

Nutritional Values: Calories: 295, Fat: 15g, Carbs: 9g, Protein: 33g, Sugar: 2g, Sodium: 125 mg, Potassium: 610 mg, Cholesterol: 85 mg

Baked Flounder with Lemon Butter Sauce

Preparation Time: 10 min
Cooking Time: 12 min
Mode of Cooking: Baking
Servings: 4
Ingredients:

- 4 flounder fillets, 5 oz each
- 4 Tbsp butter
- 1 lemon, juiced and zested
- 2 Tbsp capers
- 1 Tbsp parsley, chopped
- 2 cloves garlic, minced
- Salt and pepper to taste

Directions:

1. Preheat oven to 350°F (177°C)
2. Place flounder fillets in a baking dish
3. In a saucepan, melt butter over medium heat, add garlic, lemon juice, lemon zest, and capers
4. Pour the lemon butter sauce over flounder and season with salt and pepper
5. Bake for 12 min or until flounder is flaky

Tips:

- Pour sauce over flounder again before serving to enhance flavor
- Pair this dish with wild rice for added texture and nutritional benefits

Nutritional Values: Calories: 216, Fat: 12g, Carbs: 3g, Protein: 24g, Sugar: 1g, Sodium: 180 mg, Potassium: 450 mg, Cholesterol: 85 mg

Mediterranean Herb-Grilled Salmon

Preparation Time: 20 min.
Cooking Time: 10 min.
Mode of Cooking: Grilling
Servings: 4
Ingredients:

- 4 salmon fillets, about 6 oz. each
- 3 Tbsp extra virgin olive oil
- 2 cloves garlic, minced
- 1 Tbsp fresh rosemary, chopped
- 1 Tbsp fresh thyme, chopped
- 1 Tbsp fresh oregano, chopped
- Juice of 1 lemon
- Salt and black pepper to taste

Directions:

1. Preheat grill to medium-high heat, around 375°F (190°C)
2. In a small bowl, combine olive oil, garlic, rosemary, thyme, oregano, lemon juice, salt, and black pepper
3. Brush the herb mixture over the salmon fillets ensuring an even coat
4. Place salmon on grill, skin-side down, and cook for about 5 min.
5. Flip carefully and grill for another 5 min. or until cooked through and flaky

Tips:

- Ensure the grill is well-oiled to prevent sticking
- Serve with a side of grilled asparagus or a fresh Mediterranean salad

Nutritional Values: Calories: 280, Fat: 18g, Carbs: 1g, Protein: 29g, Sugar: 0g, Sodium: 75 mg, Potassium: 700 mg, Cholesterol: 70 mg

Soups and Stews with Seafood

Lemongrass Shrimp and Coconut Soup

Preparation Time: 20 min.
Cooking Time: 30 min.
Mode of Cooking: Simmering
Servings: 4
Ingredients:

- 1 Tbsp olive oil
- 2 stalks lemongrass, minced

- 1 inch ginger, peeled and grated
- 4 cups chicken broth
- 1 can (14 oz.) coconut milk
- 1 lb. shrimp, peeled and deveined
- 1 cup mushrooms, thinly sliced
- 1 red bell pepper, julienned
- 1 Tbsp fish sauce
- Juice of 1 lime
- 1 tsp coconut sugar
- Cilantro and fresh chili slices, for garnish

Directions:

1. Heat olive oil in a large pot over medium heat
2. Add minced lemongrass and grated ginger, sauté until fragrant, about 3 min.
3. Pour in chicken broth and coconut milk, bring to a simmer
4. Add shrimp, mushrooms, and red bell pepper, cook until shrimp are pink and vegetables are tender, about 10 min.
5. Stir in fish sauce, lime juice, and coconut sugar
6. Serve garnished with cilantro and fresh chili slices

Tips:

- Use fresh lemongrass for the best flavor
- Add chili slices according to spice preference

Nutritional Values: Calories: 250, Fat: 15g, Carbs: 10g, Protein: 20g, Sugar: 3g, Sodium: 850 mg, Potassium: 300 mg, Cholesterol: 120 mg

Saffron Tomato Bouillabaisse

Preparation Time: 15 min.
Cooking Time: 45 min.
Mode of Cooking: Boiling
Servings: 6
Ingredients:

- 2 Tbsp olive oil
- 1 fennel bulb, chopped
- 1 onion, chopped
- 3 cloves garlic, minced
- Pinch of saffron threads
- 1 quart vegetable stock
- 1 can (28 oz.) crushed tomatoes
- 1 lb. mixed seafood (clams, mussels, shrimp, and fish pieces)
- 1 Tbsp fresh parsley, chopped
- Zest of one orange
- Salt and pepper to taste

Directions:

1. In a large pot, heat olive oil over medium heat
2. Add fennel, onion, and garlic, cook until softened, about 7 min.
3. Add saffron, then pour in vegetable stock and crushed tomatoes, bring to a boil
4. Add mixed seafood, cover, and simmer until shellfish open and fish is cooked through, about 25 min.
5. Stir in fresh parsley and orange zest
6. Season with salt and pepper before serving

Tips:

- Discard any shellfish that do not open after cooking
- Serve with crusty bread for dipping
- Saffron lends a luxurious flavor and color to the dish

Nutritional Values: Calories: 180, Fat: 5g, Carbs: 12g, Protein: 22g, Sugar: 4g, Sodium: 700 mg, Potassium: 450 mg, Cholesterol: 85 mg

Cod and Potato Stew

Preparation Time: 10 min.
Cooking Time: 35 min.
Mode of Cooking: Simmering
Servings: 4
Ingredients:

- 1 Tbsp extra virgin olive oil
- 2 cloves garlic, minced
- 1 onion, chopped
- 2 carrots, sliced
- 2 potatoes, cubed
- 4 cups fish stock
- 1 lb. cod fillets, cut into chunks
- 1 tsp dried thyme
- Salt and pepper to taste
- Chopped parsley for garnish

Directions:

1. In a large pot, heat olive oil over medium heat
2. Add garlic, onion, and carrots, sauté until onions are translucent, about 5 min.

3. Add potatoes and fish stock, bring to a simmer and cook until potatoes are tender, about 20 min.
4. Add cod fillets and thyme, cook until fish flakes easily with a fork, about 10 min.
5. Season with salt and pepper
6. Garnish with parsley before serving

Tips:

- Choose firm potatoes that hold their shape well during cooking
- This stew can be thickened with a roux if preferred
- Fresh herbs may be added for extra flavor

Nutritional Values: Calories: 220, Fat: 5g, Carbs: 18g, Protein: 25g, Sugar: 3g, Sodium: 670 mg, Potassium: 800 mg, Cholesterol: 60 mg

Spicy Miso Seafood Soup

Preparation Time: 15 min.
Cooking Time: 25 min.
Mode of Cooking: Simmering
Servings: 4
Ingredients:

- 2 Tbsp miso paste
- 4 cups water
- 1 Tbsp sesame oil
- 1 tsp chili flakes
- 1 lb. assorted seafood (shrimp, scallops, squid)
- 1 cup shiitake mushrooms, sliced
- 2 scallions, chopped
- 1 Tbsp soy sauce
- 1 tsp grated ginger
- 1 small bunch of bok choy, chopped

Directions:

1. In a pot, dissolve miso paste in water over medium heat and bring to a simmer
2. In a separate pan, heat sesame oil and chili flakes for 2 min.
3. Add seafood and stir-fry until just cooked, about 5 min.
4. Transfer seafood to the miso broth
5. Add shiitake mushrooms, scallions, soy sauce, ginger, and bok choy
6. Simmer for 10 min.
7. Adjust seasoning as needed

Tips:

- Do not boil the miso broth as it can affect the flavor and nutritional value
- Add tofu for an extra protein boost
- Adjust chili flakes according to spice tolerance

Nutritional Values: Calories: 180, Fat: 8g, Carbs: 9g, Protein: 20g, Sugar: 2g, Sodium: 900 mg, Potassium: 350 mg, Cholesterol: 95 mg

Herb-Infused Fish Stew

Preparation Time: 20 min.
Cooking Time: 40 min.
Mode of Cooking: Braising
Servings: 6
Ingredients:

- 3 Tbsp olive oil
- 1 cup leeks, white and light green parts only, sliced
- 2 cloves garlic, minced
- 1 cup dry white wine
- 1 qt. fish stock
- 2 tomatoes, diced
- 1 lb. firm white fish, like halibut, cut into large pieces
- 1 Tbsp chopped fresh basil
- 1 Tbsp chopped fresh dill
- Salt and pepper to taste

Directions:

1. Heat olive oil in a large pot over medium heat
2. Add leeks and garlic, cook until leeks are softened, about 8 min.
3. Pour in white wine, reduce by half
4. Add fish stock and tomatoes, bring to a simmer
5. Carefully place fish pieces into the pot, cover and simmer gently until fish is cooked, about 20 min.
6. Stir in fresh basil and dill
7. Season with salt and pepper before serving

Tips:

- Use fresh herbs for the best flavor and aroma
- If desired, add clams or mussels during the last 10 min. of cooking for variety
- Serve with a drizzle of quality extra virgin olive oil for enhanced richness

Nutritional Values: Calories: 210, Fat: 10g, Carbs: 5g, Protein: 23g, Sugar: 2g, Sodium: 860 mg, Potassium: 500 mg, Cholesterol: 60 mg

Mediterranean Monkfish Stew

Preparation Time: 15 min
Cooking Time: 35 min
Mode of Cooking: Simmering
Servings: 4
Ingredients:

- 2 lb. monkfish, cubed
- 3 Tbsp extra virgin olive oil
- 1 large onion, chopped
- 4 garlic cloves, minced
- 1 bell pepper, diced
- 1 fennel bulb, thinly sliced
- 14 oz. can diced tomatoes
- 1 tsp saffron threads
- 1 qt. fish stock
- ½ cup dry white wine
- ¼ cup fresh parsley, chopped
- Salt to taste
- Black pepper to taste

Directions:

1. Heat olive oil in a large pot over medium heat
2. Add onion and garlic, sauté until soft
3. Mix in bell pepper and fennel, cook until slightly tender
4. Stir in tomatoes, saffron, fish stock, and white wine, bring to a boil
5. Reduce heat, add monkfish, simmer for 25 min
6. Season with salt and black pepper, sprinkle with parsley before serving

Tips:

- Use fresh saffron for a more intense flavor
- Pair with a slice of whole-grain bread to soak up the broth
- If monkfish is unavailable, substitute with another firm white fish

Nutritional Values: Calories: 310, Fat: 10g, Carbs: 16g, Protein: 36g, Sugar: 5g, Sodium: 620 mg, Potassium: 840 mg, Cholesterol: 85 mg

Quick Seafood Recipes for Busy Evenings

Lemon Garlic Shrimp with Zucchini Noodles

Preparation Time: 15 min
Cooking Time: 10 min
Mode of Cooking: Sautéing
Servings: 4
Ingredients:

- 1 lb shrimp, peeled and deveined
- 2 large zucchinis, spiralized
- 3 Tbsp olive oil
- 4 cloves garlic, minced
- 1 lemon, juiced and zested
- 1 tsp red pepper flakes
- Salt and pepper to taste
- Fresh parsley, chopped for garnish

Directions:

1. Heat 2 Tbsp of olive oil over medium-high heat
2. Add minced garlic and red pepper flakes, sauté for 1 min
3. Add shrimp and sauté until pink and cooked through, about 6-7 min, turning occasionally
4. Remove shrimp and set aside
5. In the same pan, add remaining 1 Tbsp olive oil and spiralized zucchini, sauté for about 3 minutes until tender
6. Return shrimp to pan, add lemon juice and zest, toss to combine
7. Season with salt and pepper, garnish with parsley

Tips:

- Serve immediately for best texture of zucchini noodles
- Use wild-caught shrimp for richer flavor and nutritional benefits

Nutritional Values: Calories: 240, Fat: 10g, Carbs: 6g, Protein: 32g, Sugar: 2g, Sodium: 470 mg, Potassium: 300 mg, Cholesterol: 182 mg

Spicy Tuna Tartare Stacks

Preparation Time: 20 min
Cooking Time: none
Mode of Cooking: Arranging
Servings: 4
Ingredients:

- 8 oz. ahi tuna, finely diced
- 1 ripe avocado, diced
- 1/2 cucumber, diced
- 2 Tbsp sesame oil
- 1 Tbsp soy sauce
- 1 tsp wasabi paste
- 1 tsp ginger, grated
- 1 Tbsp black sesame seeds
- Salt to taste

Directions:

1. Combine soy sauce, sesame oil, wasabi, and ginger in a bowl
2. Add tuna, avocado, and cucumber to the sauce mixture and gently toss to coat
3. Plate the mixture using a round mold, layering tuna at the bottom, followed by avocado and cucumber on top
4. Gently remove the mold and sprinkle with black sesame seeds. Season with salt

Tips:

- Serve immediately to maintain freshness of the tuna
- Use gluten-free soy sauce for a gluten-sensitive diet
- Pair with a chilled glass of dry white wine for an elegant touch

Nutritional Values: Calories: 190, Fat: 10g, Carbs: 5g, Protein: 20g, Sugar: 1g, Sodium: 320 mg, Potassium: 500 mg, Cholesterol: 30 mg

Broiled Tilapia with Mustard-Chive Sauce

Preparation Time: 10 min
Cooking Time: 15 min
Mode of Cooking: Broiling
Servings: 4
Ingredients:

- 4 tilapia fillets
- 2 Tbsp Dijon mustard
- 1/4 cup Greek yogurt
- 1/4 cup chives, finely chopped
- 1 lemon, juiced
- 2 Tbsp olive oil
- Salt and pepper to taste
- Lemon wedges for serving

Directions:

1. Preheat broiler to 400°F (200°C)
2. Arrange tilapia fillets on a greased baking sheet
3. In a bowl, mix together mustard, Greek yogurt, lemon juice, and chives
4. Brush fillets with olive oil, season with salt and pepper
5. Spoon mustard-chive mixture over each fillet
6. Broil for about 10-12 min until fish flakes easily with a fork

Tips:

- Serve with lemon wedges and a side of steamed asparagus
- This dressing can also be used with salmon or cod

Nutritional Values: Calories: 180, Fat: 9g, Carbs: 2g, Protein: 23g, Sugar: 1g, Sodium: 125 mg, Potassium: 460 mg, Cholesterol: 55 mg

Scallop Ceviche with Mango and Avocado

Preparation Time: 30 min
Cooking Time: none
Mode of Cooking: Marinating
Servings: 4
Ingredients:

- 12 large scallops, thinly sliced
- 1 ripe mango, diced
- 1 avocado, diced
- 1 small red onion, finely chopped
- 1 jalapeño, seeded and minced
- Juice of 2 limes
- 1/4 cup fresh cilantro, chopped
- Salt and pepper to taste

Directions:

1. Combine lime juice, red onion, and jalapeño in a large bowl
2. Add scallops to the lime mixture and allow to marinate in the refrigerator for about 20 min

3. Just before serving, add mango, avocado, and cilantro to the scallops
4. Season with salt and pepper and mix gently

Tips:

- Serve immediately after preparation to enjoy the freshness of the seafood
- Serve in individual glasses for a visually appealing presentation
- Drizzle with a bit of extra-virgin olive oil to enhance flavors

Nutritional Values: Calories: 210, Fat: 8g, Carbs: 20g, Protein: 17g, Sugar: 7g, Sodium: 400 mg, Potassium: 470 mg, Cholesterol: 27 mg

Quick Garlic Butter Cod with Parsley

Preparation Time: 10 min
Cooking Time: 15 min
Mode of Cooking: Pan-frying
Servings: 4

Ingredients:

- 4 cod fillets
- 4 Tbsp unsalted butter
- 4 cloves garlic, minced
- Juice of 1 lemon
- 1/4 cup fresh parsley, chopped
- Salt and pepper to taste
- Lemon slices for garnish

Directions:

1. Heat butter in a large skillet over medium heat
2. Add minced garlic and sauté until fragrant, about 1 min
3. Place cod fillets in the skillet and season with salt and pepper
4. Cook for about 6-7 min on each side until cooked through and golden
5. Drizzle with lemon juice, sprinkle with chopped parsley

Tips:

- Serve with steamed green beans and garnish with lemon slices
- Use paper towels to pat dry cod fillets before cooking to avoid excess moisture and achieve a better sear

Nutritional Values: Calories: 220, Fat: 14g, Carbs: 2g, Protein: 23g, Sugar: 0g, Sodium: 85 mg, Potassium: 520 mg, Cholesterol: 60 mg

Lemon and Dill Haddock Parcels

Preparation Time: 10 min.
Cooking Time: 12 min.
Mode of Cooking: Baking
Servings: 2

Ingredients:

- 2 haddock fillets, about 6 oz. each
- 1 lemon, thinly sliced
- 2 sprigs fresh dill
- 1 Tbsp extra virgin olive oil
- 1 tsp garlic, minced
- Salt to taste
- Black pepper to taste

Directions:

1. Preheat oven to 375°F (190°C)
2. Lay out two sheets of aluminum foil, place a haddock fillet on each
3. Season fish with salt, black pepper, and minced garlic
4. Top each fillet with lemon slices and a sprig of dill
5. Drizzle with olive oil
6. Wrap the foil around the fish, sealing the edges tightly to form parcels
7. Bake in the preheated oven for about 12 min.

Tips:

- Always ensure the foil is tightly sealed to keep moisture in
- Serve immediately to enjoy the full flavor of the herbs and lemon

Nutritional Values: Calories: 190, Fat: 7g, Carbs: 2g, Protein: 28g, Sugar: 1g, Sodium: 125 mg, Potassium: 500 mg, Cholesterol: 70 mg

9.Main Dishes: Poultry Recipes

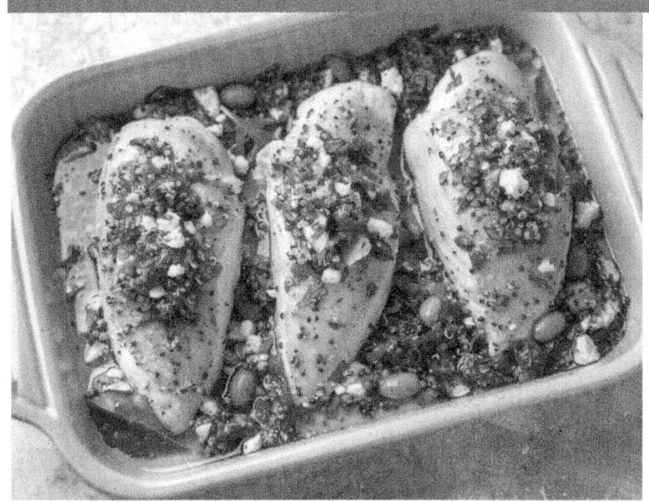

As we journey deeper into the heart of balanced nutrition tailored for menopause, it's time to turn our attention to a cornerstone of wholesome diets: poultry. Often lauded for its versatility and lean protein content, poultry acts not only as a culinary hero but also as a stalwart ally in our quest for hormonal equilibrium and weight management during this transformative period of life.

In structuring this chapter, I aim to guide you through an exploration of chicken and turkey recipes that will not only nurture your body but also delight your taste buds. These aren't your average poultry dishes; each recipe is crafted with an eye towards combating inflammation and supporting a healthy metabolic rate, which can sometimes slow down during menopause.

Picture this: a Sunday family dinner, the table set with a golden, roasted chicken seasoned with herbs that not only tantalize the palate but also confer health benefits like improved digestion and reduced stress levels. Or imagine a quick weekday night, where you transform some simple turkey leftovers into a vibrant, aromatic stir-fry that keeps you feeling light and energetic, ready to take on the next day's challenges.

This chapter focuses on making poultry a central part of your diet, aligning with our overall goals of managing menopause symptoms through food. We'll explore ways to prepare chicken and turkey not just as mere ingredients, but as exciting, flavorful elements of hearty meals that your family will request time and again. From comforting soups that soothe the soul to one-pot wonders that simplify your meal preparation, each dish serves a purpose more significant than satiety alone.

Whether you're looking to revamp your culinary routine or find solace in new, health-boosting recipes, this poultry chapter promises to elevate your cooking repertoire, making each meal an opportunity to nourish both body and spirit during a pivotal time of your life. Let's embrace the flavors and potentials that these wholesome dishes have to offer!

Homestyle Chicken Recipes

Mediterranean Stuffed Chicken Breasts

Preparation Time: 20 min

Cooking Time: 45 min

Mode of Cooking: Baking

Servings: 4

Ingredients:

- 4 boneless chicken breasts
- 1 cup cooked quinoa
- ½ cup sun-dried tomatoes, chopped
- ½ cup kalamata olives, pitted and chopped
- 1 cup spinach, chopped
- ½ cup feta cheese, crumbled
- 3 cloves garlic, minced
- 2 Tbsp extra virgin olive oil
- 1 tsp dried basil
- 1 tsp dried oregano
- Salt and pepper to taste

Directions:

1. Preheat oven to 375°F (190°C)
2. In a bowl, mix quinoa, sun-dried tomatoes, olives, spinach, feta, garlic, basil, and oregano
3. Cut a pocket horizontally into each chicken breast and stuff with the quinoa mixture
4. Secure with toothpicks if necessary
5. Season the outside of the chicken with salt, pepper, and drizzle with olive oil

6. Place in a baking dish and bake for 45 min or until chicken is thoroughly cooked and juices run clear

Tips:

- Consider using toothpicks to secure the stuffing inside the chicken during baking
- Serve with a side of mixed greens for a complete meal
- Leftovers can be sliced and added to salads or wraps

Nutritional Values: Calories: 415, Fat: 19g, Carbs: 22g, Protein: 38g, Sugar: 3g, Sodium: 620 mg, Potassium: 407 mg, Cholesterol: 105 mg

Herb-Encrusted Chicken Parmesan

Preparation Time: 15 min
Cooking Time: 30 min
Mode of Cooking: Grilling and Baking
Servings: 4
Ingredients:

- 4 boneless chicken breasts
- 1 cup whole wheat breadcrumbs
- ½ cup Parmesan cheese, grated
- 1 Tbsp Italian seasoning
- 3 Tbsp olive oil
- 1 cup tomato sauce, no sugar added
- 1 cup shredded mozzarella cheese
- Salt and pepper to taste
- Fresh basil leaves for garnish

Directions:

1. Preheat oven to 375°F (190°C)
2. Mix breadcrumbs, Parmesan cheese, and Italian seasoning in a bowl
3. Brush each chicken breast with olive oil, then dredge in breadcrumb mixture
4. Preheat grill or grill pan over medium heat, grill chicken for 3-4 min on each side until golden
5. Place grilled chicken in a baking dish, top each with tomato sauce and mozzarella cheese
6. Bake in oven for 20-25 min until cheese is bubbly and chicken is cooked through

Tips:

- Use whole wheat breadcrumbs for added fiber
- Garnish with fresh basil leaves before serving for enhanced flavor
- Pair with a vegetable salad for a balanced meal

Nutritional Values: Calories: 390, Fat: 18g, Carbs: 19g, Protein: 40g, Sugar: 4g, Sodium: 620 mg, Potassium: 300 mg, Cholesterol: 98 mg

Lemon Thyme Chicken Skillet

Preparation Time: 10 min
Cooking Time: 20 min
Mode of Cooking: Sautéing
Servings: 4
Ingredients:

- 4 chicken thighs, bone-in, skin-on
- 1 lemon, sliced
- 4 cloves garlic, minced
- 1 cup chicken broth
- 2 Tbsp fresh thyme leaves
- 3 Tbsp olive oil
- Salt and pepper to taste

Directions:

1. Heat olive oil in a large skillet over medium-high heat
2. Season chicken thighs with salt and pepper, place them skin-side down in skillet, cook until skin is crisp, about 7 min
3. Flip chicken thighs, add garlic, lemon slices, thyme, and chicken broth
4. Reduce heat to low and cover skillet, let simmer for 13 min or until chicken is thoroughly cooked

Tips:

- To enhance the lemon flavor, add zest of one lemon to the skillet before covering
- Serve with a side of steamed asparagus or green beans
- Perfect for a quick weeknight dinner

Nutritional Values: Calories: 340, Fat: 24g, Carbs: 5g, Protein: 24g, Sugar: 1g, Sodium: 420 mg, Potassium: 334 mg, Cholesterol: 142 mg

Chicken and Shiitake Mushroom Stir-Fry

Preparation Time: 15 min
Cooking Time: 10 min
Mode of Cooking: Stir-Frying
Servings: 4
Ingredients:

- 1 lb chicken breast, thinly sliced
- 2 cups shiitake mushrooms, sliced
- 1 bell pepper, julienne
- 1 onion, sliced
- 2 Tbsp soy sauce, low sodium
- 1 Tbsp sesame oil
- 2 tsp ginger, minced
- 2 cloves garlic, minced
- 1 Tbsp cornstarch
- ¼ cup water
- 2 Tbsp olive oil
- Salt and pepper to taste

Directions:

1. Heat olive oil in a large skillet or wok over high heat
2. Add chicken and stir-fry until nearly cooked, about 4 min
3. Add mushrooms, bell pepper, onion, garlic, and ginger, continue to stir-fry for 3 min
4. Mix soy sauce, sesame oil, cornstarch, and water in a small bowl, add to the skillet, stir well to coat all ingredients, cook for 3 min or until sauce has thickened and chicken is fully cooked

Tips:

- To achieve the best texture, do not overcrowd the skillet; cook in batches if necessary
- Serve hot, ideally over a bed of cooked quinoa or brown rice
- Garnish with sesame seeds for an added crunch

Nutritional Values: Calories: 285, Fat: 12g, Carbs: 14g, Protein: 28g, Sugar: 4g, Sodium: 530 mg, Potassium: 448 mg, Cholesterol: 65 mg

Smoky Paprika Chicken Casserole

Preparation Time: 20 min

Cooking Time: 1 hr

Mode of Cooking: Baking

Servings: 6

Ingredients:

- 3 lb chicken drumsticks
- 1 can diced tomatoes
- 1 can black beans, rinsed and drained
- 1 red onion, sliced
- 2 carrots, sliced
- 1 cup chicken broth
- 2 Tbsp smoked paprika
- 3 cloves garlic, minced
- 2 Tbsp olive oil
- Salt and pepper to taste

Directions:

1. Preheat oven to 350°F (175°C)
2. In a large bowl, toss chicken drumsticks with smoked paprika, garlic, salt, and pepper
3. Heat olive oil in a large skillet, brown drumsticks over medium-high heat, about 3 min each side
4. Transfer drumsticks to a large casserole dish, add diced tomatoes, black beans, red onion, carrots, and chicken broth
5. Cover and bake in the oven for 1 hr or until chicken is tender

Tips:

- Adding a touch of honey to the casserole can balance the smokiness of the paprika
- Perfect to serve with rustic bread or mashed potatoes
- Leftovers can be stored in the refrigerator for up to 3 days and make great fillings for wraps or sandwiches

Nutritional Values: Calories: 290, Fat: 15g, Carbs: 18g, Protein: 22g, Sugar: 5g, Sodium: 410 mg, Potassium: 530 mg, Cholesterol: 82 mg

Mediterranean Stuffed Chicken

Preparation Time: 20 min.

Cooking Time: 25 min.

Mode of Cooking: Baking

Servings: 4

Ingredients:

- 4 boneless, skinless chicken breasts
- 1 cup fresh spinach, chopped
- ½ cup feta cheese, crumbled
- ¼ cup sun-dried tomatoes, chopped
- 2 cloves garlic, minced
- 1 Tbsp olive oil
- 1 tsp dried oregano
- Salt and pepper to taste

Directions:

1. Preheat oven to 375°F (190°C)

2. Make a horizontal cut through the thickest part of each chicken breast to form a pocket
3. Mix spinach, feta, sun-dried tomatoes, garlic, and oregano in a bowl
4. Stuff each chicken breast with the mixture and secure with toothpicks
5. Season with salt and pepper
6. Heat olive oil in a skillet over medium heat and sear chicken on both sides until golden
7. Transfer to a baking dish and bake in the oven for 20 minutes or until chicken is cooked through

Tips:

- Allow chicken to rest for 5 minutes before serving to retain juices
- Serve with a side of quinoa or a fresh salad to keep the meal light and balanced

Nutritional Values: Calories: 290, Fat: 13g, Carbs: 8g, Protein: 35g, Sugar: 3g, Sodium: 400 mg, Potassium: 500 mg, Cholesterol: 105 mg

EXPLORING TURKEY BEYOND HOLIDAY MEALS

TURKEY PICCATA WITH CITRUS ACCENTS

Preparation Time: 15 min.
Cooking Time: 20 min.
Mode of Cooking: Sautéing
Servings: 4
Ingredients:

- 4 turkey breast cutlets, pounded thin
- ½ cup almond flour
- 1 tsp garlic powder
- Salt and pepper to taste
- 2 Tbsp olive oil
- 1/4 cup freshly squeezed lemon juice
- 1/2 cup chicken broth
- 1/4 cup capers, drained
- Zest of 1 orange
- 2 Tbsp fresh parsley, chopped
- 1 Tbsp unsalted butter

Directions:

1. Season turkey cutlets with garlic powder, salt, and pepper and dredge in almond flour
2. Heat olive oil in a pan over medium heat and sauté cutlets until golden, about 3 min. per side
3. Remove turkey from pan
4. Add lemon juice, chicken broth, and capers to the pan, bring to a simmer, scraping up the browned bits from the pan
5. Cook until the sauce has reduced by half, about 5 min.
6. Stir in orange zest and butter until butter is melted and the sauce is silky
7. Return turkey to the pan and coat with the sauce, simmering for another 2 min.
8. Garnish with fresh parsley before serving

Tips:

- Serve with a side of steamed asparagus or green beans for added nutrition
- Adjust sauce thickness by simmering for longer if desired

Nutritional Values: Calories: 310, Fat: 15g, Carbs: 8g, Protein: 35g, Sugar: 2g, Sodium: 200 mg, Potassium: 280 mg, Cholesterol: 80 mg

SMOKEY TURKEY AND LENTIL STEW

Preparation Time: 10 min.
Cooking Time: 30 min.
Mode of Cooking: Simmering
Servings: 6
Ingredients:

- 1 lb ground turkey
- 1 cup green lentils, rinsed
- 1 large onion, chopped
- 2 carrots, diced
- 1 celery stalk, diced
- 3 cloves garlic, minced
- 1 Tbsp smoked paprika
- 1 tsp ground cumin
- 2 Tbsp olive oil
- 4 cups vegetable broth
- 1 Tbsp apple cider vinegar
- Salt and pepper to taste
- Fresh cilantro for garnish

Directions:

1. Heat olive oil in a large pot over medium heat
2. Add onions, carrots, and celery, cook until onions are translucent
3. Add garlic, smoked paprika, and cumin, cook for another 1 min.
4. Add ground turkey, cook until browned
5. Stir in lentils and vegetable broth, bring to a boil
6. Reduce heat to low and simmer covered for 25 min. or until lentils are tender
7. Stir in apple cider vinegar, season with salt and pepper
8. Garnish with chopped cilantro before serving

Tips:

- Enhance flavor by adding a dash of hot sauce
- Store leftovers in the fridge for up to 3 days for a quick reheat meal

Nutritional Values: Calories: 265, Fat: 9g, Carbs: 25g, Protein: 23g, Sugar: 3g, Sodium: 300 mg, Potassium: 400 mg, Cholesterol: 55 mg

Turkish Stuffed Turkey Fillets

Preparation Time: 20 min.

Cooking Time: 25 min.

Mode of Cooking: Baking

Servings: 4

Ingredients:

- 4 turkey breast fillets, butterfly cut
- 1/2 cup fine bulgur wheat, soaked and drained
- 1 small onion, finely chopped
- 2 Tbsp pine nuts
- 1/4 cup dried currants
- 2 Tbsp fresh mint, chopped
- 1 Tbsp olive oil
- 1/2 tsp cinnamon
- Salt and pepper to taste
- 1/2 cup water

Directions:

1. Preheat oven to 375°F (190°C)
2. In a bowl, mix bulgur, onion, pine nuts, currants, mint, cinnamon, salt, and pepper

- Open turkey fillets and divide the bulgur mixture among them
- Roll up the fillets and secure with toothpicks
- Place in a baking dish and drizzle with olive oil
- Add water to the dish
- Cover with foil and bake for 20 min.

1. Remove foil and bake for an additional 5 min. or until turkey is cooked through

Tips:

- Serve these with a yogurt cucumber dip for added flavor
- Can be prepared ahead and kept in the fridge overnight

Nutritional Values: Calories: 285, Fat: 9g, Carbs: 23g, Protein: 31g, Sugar: 5g, Sodium: 65 mg, Potassium: 340 mg, Cholesterol: 70 mg

Creamy Coconut Turkey Curry

Preparation Time: 15 min.

Cooking Time: 20 min.

Mode of Cooking: Stir-frying

Servings: 4

Ingredients:

- 1 lb turkey breast, cut into cubes
- 1 Tbsp coconut oil
- 1 onion, sliced
- 2 cloves garlic, minced
- 1 Tbsp ginger, grated
- 1 Tbsp yellow curry powder
- 1 can (14 oz) coconut milk
- 1 bell pepper, chopped
- 1 cup spinach leaves
- Salt and pepper to taste
- Fresh coriander for garnish

Directions:

2. Heat coconut oil in a large skillet over medium heat
3. Add onion, garlic, and ginger, sauté until onion is soft
4. Add turkey and curry powder, cook until turkey is browned
5. Pour in coconut milk and add bell pepper

- Simmer for 10 min. until sauce thickens and bell pepper is tender

1. Stir in spinach until wilted
2. Season with salt and pepper
3. Garnish with fresh coriander before serving

Tips:

- Serve over steamed brown rice for a wholesome meal
- Add extra curry powder for a spicier flavor

Nutritional Values: Calories: 315, Fat: 22g, Carbs: 8g, Protein: 24g, Sugar: 3g, Sodium: 120 mg, Potassium: 370 mg, Cholesterol: 60 mg

AUTUMN HARVEST TURKEY CASSEROLE

Preparation Time: 20 min.

Cooking Time: 45 min.

Mode of Cooking: Baking

Servings: 6

Ingredients:

- 2 lbs turkey breast, cubed
- 1 sweet potato, peeled and diced
- 1 apple, diced
- 1/2 cup cranberries
- 1 onion, chopped
- 2 cloves garlic, minced
- 1 tsp dried thyme
- 1/2 tsp ground nutmeg
- 2 Tbsp olive oil
- 1 cup low-sodium chicken broth
- Salt and pepper to taste

Directions:

1. Preheat oven to 350°F (175°C)
2. In a large skillet, heat olive oil over medium heat
3. Add onion and garlic, cook until softened
4. Add turkey, thyme, nutmeg, salt, and pepper, cook until turkey is browned
5. In a mixing bowl, combine turkey mixture, sweet potato, apple, cranberries, and chicken broth

- Transfer to a casserole dish
- Cover and bake for 40 min.

1. Uncover and bake for an additional 5 min. to brown the top

Tips:

- Perfect served hot directly from the oven
- Sprinkle with fresh thyme before serving for extra flavor

Nutritional Values: Calories: 330, Fat: 12g, Carbs: 15g, Protein: 38g, Sugar: 8g, Sodium: 80 mg, Potassium: 490 mg, Cholesterol: 90 mg

TURKEY PICCATA WITH ARTICHOKES

Preparation Time: 20 min.

Cooking Time: 25 min.

Mode of Cooking: Sautéing

Servings: 4

Ingredients:

- 4 turkey breast cutlets, pounded thin
- 1/4 C. all-purpose flour
- 1/2 tsp. salt
- 1/4 tsp. black pepper
- 2 Tbsp. olive oil
- 1/2 C. chicken broth
- 1/4 C. fresh lemon juice
- 1 can artichoke hearts, drained and quartered
- 2 Tbsp. capers, drained
- 2 Tbsp. fresh parsley, chopped
- 1 Tbsp. unsalted butter

Directions:

2. Season turkey cutlets with salt and pepper, then dredge in flour, shaking off excess
3. Heat olive oil in a large skillet over medium-high heat and sauté turkey until golden and cooked through, about 4 min. per side
4. Remove turkey from skillet and set aside
5. In the same skillet, add chicken broth, lemon juice, and bring to a simmer
6. Stir in artichoke hearts and capers, and simmer for 5 min.
7. Return turkey to skillet and warm through
8. Stir in butter and parsley just before serving

Tips:

- Serve with a side of steamed vegetables or a fresh garden salad for a complete meal
- Capers can be substituted with diced olives for a twist

Nutritional Values: Calories: 295, Fat: 12g, Carbs: 17g, Protein: 28g, Sugar: 1g, Sodium: 580 mg, Potassium: 300 mg, Cholesterol: 70 mg

TURMERIC & GINGER CHICKEN STEW

Preparation Time: 20 min
Cooking Time: 40 min
Mode of Cooking: Stovetop
Servings: 4
Ingredients:

- 2 lb. chicken thighs, boneless and skinless
- 1 large onion, finely chopped
- 3 cloves garlic, minced
- 2 Tbsp fresh ginger, grated
- 1 tsp turmeric powder
- 1 tsp ground cumin
- 1 can (14 oz.) coconut milk
- 2 Tbsp olive oil
- 1 cup chicken broth
- 2 carrots, sliced
- 1 bell pepper, chopped
- Salt and pepper to taste
- Fresh cilantro, chopped for garnish

Directions:

1. Heat olive oil in a large pot over medium heat. Add onion, garlic, and ginger and sauté until onion is translucent
2. Stir in turmeric, cumin, salt, and pepper, and cook for 1 min
3. Add chicken thighs and brown evenly on both sides
4. Pour in coconut milk and chicken broth, bring to a simmer
5. Add carrots and bell pepper, cover, and simmer on low heat for 35 min
6. Garnish with fresh cilantro before serving

Tips:

- Serve with a side of quinoa for a complete meal
- Ideal for prepping ahead and tastes even better the next day

Nutritional Values: Calories: 480, Fat: 29g, Carbs: 13g, Protein: 40g, Sugar: 5g, Sodium: 300 mg, Potassium: 650 mg, Cholesterol: 120 mg

LEMON & THYME BRAISED CHICKEN

Preparation Time: 15 min
Cooking Time: 1 hr
Mode of Cooking: Stovetop
Servings: 6
Ingredients:

- 3 lb. chicken pieces (thighs and breasts)
- 1 lemon, thinly sliced
- 4 sprigs fresh thyme
- 3 Tbsp extra virgin olive oil
- 1 cup low-sodium chicken broth
- 1 bulb fennel, thinly sliced
- 2 leeks, white and light green parts sliced
- Salt and pepper to taste
- 1 Tbsp whole grain mustard

Directions:

1. Preheat a large skillet with olive oil over medium-high heat
2. Season chicken with salt and pepper and brown on all sides
3. Remove chicken and add leeks and fennel to the skillet, sauté until soft
4. Return chicken to the skillet, add lemon slices, thyme, and chicken broth
5. Cover and simmer on low heat for about 50 min
6. Stir in whole grain mustard before serving

Tips:

- Perfect paired with a steamy bowl of bulgur or brown rice
- Can be stored and reheated, maintaining its flavors and tenderness

Nutritional Values: Calories: 410, Fat: 24g, Carbs: 9g, Protein: 35g, Sugar: 3g, Sodium: 200 mg, Potassium: 380 mg, Cholesterol: 105 mg

SPICY TOMATO AND CHICKEN RAGOUT

Preparation Time: 25 min
Cooking Time: 1 hr
Mode of Cooking: Stovetop
Servings: 4
Ingredients:

- 2 lb. chicken drumsticks

- 1 large can (28 oz.) crushed tomatoes
- 1 onion, diced
- 3 cloves garlic, minced
- 2 Tbsp smoked paprika
- 1 tsp chili flakes
- 2 Tbsp olive oil
- 1 cup low-sodium chicken broth
- 1 red bell pepper, diced
- 1 zucchini, diced
- Salt and pepper to taste
- Parsley, chopped for garnish

Directions:

1. Heat olive oil in a pot over medium heat
2. Add onion and garlic and cook until softened
3. Stir in smoked paprika, chili flakes, and season with salt and pepper
4. Add chicken drumsticks and sear until all sides are lightly browned
5. Pour in crushed tomatoes and chicken broth, bring to a boil
6. Reduce heat to a simmer, add bell pepper and zucchini, and cook covered for 50 min
7. Garnish with chopped parsley before serving

Tips:

- A robust dish that benefits from overnight resting, enhancing its flavors
- Complements a rustic loaf of bread for sopping up the hearty sauce

Nutritional Values: Calories: 350, Fat: 15g, Carbs: 24g, Protein: 25g, Sugar: 8g, Sodium: 220 mg, Potassium: 800 mg, Cholesterol: 80 mg

Chicken and Mushroom Cream Stew

Preparation Time: 15 min

Cooking Time: 30 min

Mode of Cooking: Stovetop

Servings: 5

Ingredients:

- 1 lb. chicken breasts, cubed
- 1 lb. mushrooms, sliced
- 3 Tbsp unsalted butter
- 2 Tbsp whole wheat flour
- 1 cup skim milk
- 1 cup low-sodium chicken broth
- 2 onions, chopped
- 3 cloves garlic, minced
- 1 Tbsp fresh tarragon, chopped
- Salt and pepper to taste

Directions:

1. Melt butter in a large pot over medium heat
2. Add onions and garlic, cooking until onions are translucent
3. Stir in flour and cook for 2 min
4. Gradually add milk and chicken broth, whisking to prevent lumps
5. Add chicken and mushrooms, bring to a simmer and cook until chicken is cooked through, about 25 min
6. Season with salt, pepper, and tarragon before serving

Tips:

- Can be thickened with more flour for a creamier texture
- Pairs beautifully with steamed rice or a baked potato

Nutritional Values: Calories: 310, Fat: 12g, Carbs: 18g, Protein: 29g, Sugar: 7g, Sodium: 150 mg, Potassium: 690 mg, Cholesterol: 75 mg

Moroccan Lemon Chicken Tagine

Preparation Time: 20 min

Cooking Time: 1 hr 10 min

Mode of Cooking: Slow Cooking

Servings: 4

Ingredients:

- 2 lb. chicken thighs, boneless and skinless
- 1 onion, chopped
- 2 carrots, sliced
- 2 cloves garlic, minced
- 1 lemon, preserved and sliced
- 2 tsp ground cumin
- 1 tsp ground cinnamon
- 4 Tbsp olive oil
- 1 cup water
- 1 cup green olives, pitted
- Salt and pepper to taste
- Fresh coriander, chopped for garnish

Directions:

1. Heat olive oil in a tagine or heavy pot over medium heat

2. Add onions, garlic, and spices, cooking until onions are soft
3. Add chicken and brown on all sides
4. Incorporate preserved lemon, carrots, water, and bring to a simmer
5. Cover and cook on low heat for 60 min
6. Stir in olives and simmer for an additional 10 min
7. Garnish with fresh coriander

Tips:

- Serve with couscous to absorb the flavorful sauce
- Adjust seasoning with additional lemon or spices according to taste

Nutritional Values: Calories: 420, Fat: 26g, Carbs: 15g, Protein: 32g, Sugar: 5g, Sodium: 620 mg, Potassium: 430 mg, Cholesterol: 140 mg

Tuscan Chicken Stew

Preparation Time: 15 min
Cooking Time: 1 hr
Mode of Cooking: Simmering
Servings: 4
Ingredients:

- 2 lb chicken thighs, boneless and skinless
- 1 large onion, finely chopped
- 3 garlic cloves, minced
- 1 red bell pepper, diced
- 2 carrots, sliced
- 1 zucchini, sliced
- 14 oz canned diced tomatoes
- 2 Tbsp tomato paste
- 4 cups chicken broth
- 1 Tbsp Italian seasoning
- 1 tsp dried basil
- Salt and pepper to taste
- 2 Tbsp olive oil

Directions:

1. Heat olive oil in a large pot over medium heat
2. Add onion and garlic, sauté until soft
3. Add chicken thighs, brown on each side for 4-5 min
4. Add bell pepper, carrots, zucchini, diced tomatoes, tomato paste, chicken broth, Italian seasoning, and dried basil, bring to a boil
5. Reduce heat and simmer for 1 hr, stirring occasionally

Tips:

- To thicken the stew, mash some of the vegetables softly with the back of a ladle
- Serve with whole-grain bread for added fiber
- Add a pinch of chili flakes for a spicy kick

Nutritional Values: Calories: 450, Fat: 22g, Carbs: 18g, Protein: 40g, Sugar: 12g, Sodium: 800 mg, Potassium: 650 mg, Cholesterol: 120 mg

10.Creative Sides and Appetizers

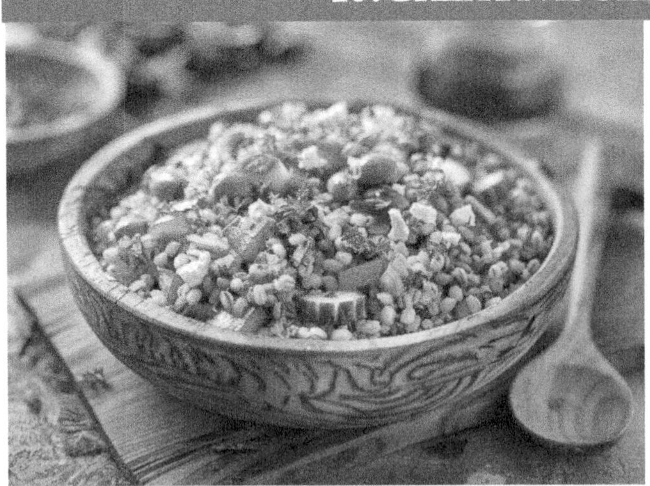

As we journey through the transformative phase of menopause, we often find comfort and delight in the smaller servings on our plate—those creative sides and appetizers that not only satisfy our palates but also provide crucial nutritional benefits. Far from being mere accompaniments or afterthoughts, these dishes play a pivotal role in maintaining our hormonal balance and fortifying our bodies against inflammation, a common adversary during menopause.

Imagine an evening surrounded by loved ones: laughter fills the air, and the table is adorned with dishes that are as nourishing as they are delectable. This is where our culinary creativity blossoms. From zesty grain dishes that invigorate the senses to legume concoctions that are rich in both flavor and fiber, the versatility of sides and appetizers enriches our dining experience, ensuring that every meal is both satisfying and health-supportive.

One might wonder why special attention to these smaller dishes is essential during menopause. As our bodies navigate the complexities of hormonal changes, every morsel counts. The foods we choose can either exacerbate symptoms like hot flashes and mood swings or help manage them. By focusing on ingredients high in anti-inflammatory properties and low in processed elements, we can significantly influence our well-being.

Take, for example, a simple dish of roasted brussels sprouts, rich in vitamins and naturally anti-inflammatory, or a refreshing chickpea salad, bursting with fiber and plant-based protein. These dishes are not only easy to prepare but also remarkably adaptable, capable of being tailored to any dietary need or preference. As we integrate such recipes into our daily routine, they become more than just food—they are tools in our toolkit for managing menopause. Through this chapter, I invite you to explore these culinary delights not just as side dishes but as essential elements of your menopause management strategy. Whether you're looking for a burst of flavor to a weekday meal or a healthful addition to a festive gathering, the recipes and insights shared here are designed to empower and inspire you, making each meal an opportunity to enhance your health and indulge your culinary creativity. Let's embrace this chapter together, one tasty, healthful bite at a time.

Tasty Grain and Legume Dishes

Mediterranean Farro Salad

Preparation Time: 15 min

Cooking Time: 30 min

Mode of Cooking: Boiling

Servings: 4

Ingredients:

- 1 cup farro
- 3 cups water
- 1 cucumber, diced
- 1 red bell pepper, diced
- ½ cup kalamata olives, pitted and sliced
- 1 small red onion, thinly sliced
- ½ cup feta cheese crumbles
- ¼ cup fresh parsley, chopped
- 3 Tbsp extra virgin olive oil
- 2 Tbsp red wine vinegar
- 1 clove garlic, minced
- Salt to taste
- Black pepper to taste

Directions:

1. Rinse farro under cold water

2. In a saucepan, bring water to boil, add farro, reduce heat, cover, and simmer for 30 min or until farro is tender
3. Drain farro and let it cool
4. In a large bowl, combine cooled farro, cucumber, red bell pepper, kalamata olives, red onion, feta cheese, and parsley
5. Whisk together olive oil, red wine vinegar, minced garlic, salt, and black pepper in a small bowl
6. Pour dressing over salad and toss to combine thoroughly

Tips:

- Store in the fridge to enhance flavors overnight, allowing them to meld
- Serve chilled as a refreshing side dish or light main course

Nutritional Values: Calories: 320, Fat: 12g, Carbs: 45g, Protein: 9g, Sugar: 4g, Sodium: 310 mg, Potassium: 490 mg, Cholesterol: 15 mg

Curried Red Lentil Quinoa Pilaf

Preparation Time: 20 min
Cooking Time: 25 min
Mode of Cooking: Simmering
Servings: 6
Ingredients:

- 1 cup red lentils
- 1 cup quinoa, rinsed and drained
- 2 ½ cups low-sodium vegetable broth
- 1 medium carrot, diced
- 1 medium onion, finely chopped
- 2 cloves garlic, minced
- 1 Tbsp olive oil
- 2 tsp curry powder
- 1 tsp cumin
- ½ tsp turmeric
- Salt to taste
- Black pepper to taste
- 2 Tbsp chopped fresh cilantro for garnish

Directions:

1. Heat olive oil in a large pan over medium heat
2. Add onions, carrots, and garlic, sauté until onions are translucent
3. Stir in curry powder, cumin, and turmeric, cook for 1 min until fragrant
4. Add red lentils, quinoa, and vegetable broth, bring to a boil
5. Reduce heat to low, cover, and simmer for 20 min until both lentils and quinoa are tender and liquid is absorbed
6. Fluff with a fork, then season with salt and black pepper
7. Garnish with fresh cilantro before serving

Tips:

- Perfect for making in batch and reheating for quick weeknight meals
- Complements grilled vegetables or lean protein for a balanced meal

Nutritional Values: Calories: 270, Fat: 4g, Carbs: 45g, Protein: 12g, Sugar: 3g, Sodium: 30 mg, Potassium: 600 mg, Cholesterol: 0 mg

Chickpea Buckwheat Tabbouleh

Preparation Time: 10 min
Cooking Time: 15 min
Mode of Cooking: Boiling
Servings: 4
Ingredients:

- 1 cup buckwheat groats
- 2 cups water
- 1 can chickpeas, drained and rinsed
- 1 large tomato, diced
- 1 cucumber, diced
- ¼ cup fresh mint, chopped
- ¼ cup fresh parsley, chopped
- ¼ cup lemon juice
- 3 Tbsp olive oil
- Salt to taste
- Black pepper to taste

Directions:

1. In a medium saucepan, bring water to a boil and add buckwheat groats
2. Lower heat and simmer for about 10-15 min until tender
3. Drain any excess water and let cool
4. In a large mixing bowl, combine cooled buckwheat groats, chickpeas, tomato, cucumber, mint, and parsley

5. In a small bowl, whisk together lemon juice, olive oil, salt, and black pepper to create a dressing
6. Pour dressing over the buckwheat mixture and toss to coat evenly

Tips:

- Serve immediately or chill to enhance flavors
- Pairs well with grilled fish or chicken for a hearty meal

Nutritional Values: Calories: 256, Fat: 9g, Carbs: 37g, Protein: 9g, Sugar: 3g, Sodium: 200 mg, Potassium: 480 mg, Cholesterol: 0 mg

Spicy Black Bean and Barley Bowl

Preparation Time: 10 min

Cooking Time: 20 min

Mode of Cooking: Boiling

Servings: 5

Ingredients:

- 1 cup barley
- 3 cups water
- 1 can black beans, drained and rinsed
- 1 avocado, sliced
- 1 red bell pepper, diced
- 1 jalapeño, seeded and finely chopped
- Juice of 1 lime
- 2 Tbsp olive oil
- 1 tsp chili powder
- ½ tsp smoked paprika
- Salt to taste
- Fresh cilantro for garnish

Directions:

1. In a large pot, bring water to a boil and add barley
2. Reduce heat to a simmer, cover, and cook for 20 min until barley is tender
3. In a large bowl, combine cooked barley, black beans, avocado, red bell pepper, and jalapeño
4. In a small bowl, whisk together lime juice, olive oil, chili powder, smoked paprika, and salt
5. Drizzle dressing over barley mixture and toss to coat evenly
6. Garnish with fresh cilantro before serving

Tips:

- Ideal for a nutritious pack-and-go lunch
- Add a dollop of Greek yogurt for extra creaminess and protein

Nutritional Values: Calories: 340, Fat: 11g, Carbs: 54g, Protein: 11g, Sugar: 2g, Sodium: 270 mg, Potassium: 690 mg, Cholesterol: 0 mg

Sorghum and Vegetable Stir-Fry

Preparation Time: 15 min

Cooking Time: 20 min

Mode of Cooking: Stir-frying

Servings: 4

Ingredients:

- 1 cup sorghum grains
- 2 ½ cups water
- 1 Tbsp sesame oil
- 1 cup broccoli florets
- 1 cup snap peas
- 1 bell pepper, sliced
- 2 carrots, sliced
- 2 Tbsp soy sauce
- 1 Tbsp ginger, minced
- 2 cloves garlic, minced
- 2 tsp honey
- Sesame seeds for garnish

Directions:

1. Rinse sorghum grains and bring to a boil in a pot with water
2. Reduce heat to simmer, cover, and cook for 50-60 min until tender and chewy
3. In a large skillet, heat sesame oil over medium-high heat
4. Add broccoli, snap peas, bell pepper, and carrots, stir-fry for 5-7 min until crisp-tender
5. Stir in cooked sorghum, soy sauce, ginger, garlic, and honey, cook for another 2-3 min
6. Garnish with sesame seeds before serving

Tips:

- Serve hot as a main dish or side dish
- Swap honey with maple syrup for a vegan version

Nutritional Values: Calories: 300, Fat: 7g, Carbs: 53g, Protein: 9g, Sugar: 5g, Sodium: 630 mg, Potassium: 410 mg, Cholesterol: 0 mg

Quinoa Tabbouleh with Edamame

Preparation Time: 20 min

Cooking Time: 15 min

Mode of Cooking: Boiling, Mixing

Servings: 6

Ingredients:

- 1 cup quinoa
- 2 cups water
- 1 cup edamame, shelled
- 1 large cucumber, diced
- 2 medium tomatoes, diced
- 1 bunch chopped fresh parsley
- 1/4 cup chopped fresh mint
- 1/4 cup olive oil
- Juice of 2 lemons
- Salt and pepper to taste

Directions:

1. Rinse quinoa under cold water and drain
2. Bring water to a boil, add quinoa, reduce heat, cover, and simmer for 15 min until water is absorbed
3. Fluff quinoa with a fork and allow to cool
4. Combine edamame, cucumber, tomatoes, parsley, and mint in a large bowl
5. Add cooled quinoa
6. Whisk together olive oil, lemon juice, salt, and pepper, then pour over salad and mix well

Tips:

- Serve chilled or at room temperature
- Makes a great side dish or light lunch

Nutritional Values: Calories: 208, Fat: 10g, Carbs: 23g, Protein: 8g, Sugar: 4g, Sodium: 13mg, Potassium: 412mg, Cholesterol: 0mg

Unique Vegetable Accompaniments

Roasted Radishes with Tahini Yogurt Dressing

Preparation Time: 10 min.

Cooking Time: 20 min.

Mode of Cooking: Roasting

Servings: 4

Ingredients:

- 1 lb. radishes, halved
- 2 Tbsp olive oil
- 1 tsp smoked paprika
- Salt to taste
- 1 cup Greek yogurt
- 2 Tbsp tahini
- 1 Tbsp lemon juice
- 1 clove garlic, minced
- 2 Tbsp chopped parsley

Directions:

1. Preheat oven to 400°F (200°C)
2. Toss radishes in olive oil, smoked paprika, and salt
3. Arrange on a baking sheet and roast until crisp and tender
4. In a bowl, mix yogurt, tahini, lemon juice, and garlic to make dressing
5. Drizzle dressing over roasted radishes and garnish with parsley

Tips:

- For extra crispiness, let the radishes roast a few minutes longer
- You can substitute Greek yogurt with any plant-based yogurt if you prefer a dairy-free version

Nutritional Values: Calories: 90, Fat: 5g, Carbs: 8g, Protein: 4g, Sugar: 3g, Sodium: 65 mg, Potassium: 270 mg, Cholesterol: 5 mg

Spiced Cauliflower Steaks with Herb Chutney

Preparation Time: 10 min.

Cooking Time: 15 min.

Mode of Cooking: Grilling

Servings: 4

Ingredients:

- 1 large cauliflower, sliced into 4 steaks
- 2 Tbsp coconut oil
- 1 tsp turmeric powder
- 1 tsp cumin powder
- Salt and pepper to taste
- 1 cup fresh cilantro
- ½ cup fresh mint leaves

- 1 green chili, de-seeded
- 1 Tbsp lime juice
- 1 Tbsp olive oil

Directions:

1. Preheat grill to medium-high heat, about 375°F (190°C)
2. Brush cauliflower steaks with coconut oil and season with turmeric, cumin, salt, and pepper
3. Grill each side for about 7-8 min. until charred and tender
4. For the chutney, blend cilantro, mint, chili, lime juice, and olive oil until smooth
5. Serve grilled steaks with herb chutney on the side

Tips:

- Ensure the grill is hot before adding cauliflower to get a good sear
- Keep the chutney refrigerated if preparing ahead

Nutritional Values: Calories: 120, Fat: 9g, Carbs: 10g, Protein: 3g, Sugar: 3g, Sodium: 30 mg, Potassium: 450 mg, Cholesterol: 0 mg

Zesty Lime & Papaya Salad

Preparation Time: 15 min.
Cooking Time: none
Mode of Cooking: No Cooking
Servings: 4
Ingredients:

- 2 cups papaya, peeled and cubed
- 1 avocado, diced
- 1 small red onion, thinly sliced
- 1 carrot, julienned
- ¼ cup fresh lime juice
- 2 Tbsp honey
- 1 Tbsp sesame oil
- Salt and pepper to taste
- ¼ cup chopped cilantro

Directions:

1. In a large bowl, combine papaya, avocado, red onion, and carrot

- In a small bowl, whisk together lime juice, honey, sesame oil, salt, and pepper to make the dressing
- Pour the dressing over the salad and toss gently
- Sprinkle with chopped cilantro before serving

Tips:

- Serve immediately after preparing to ensure freshness and vibrant colors
- For an extra kick, add a pinch of chili flakes to the dressing

Nutritional Values: Calories: 140, Fat: 7g, Carbs: 20g, Protein: 2g, Sugar: 12g, Sodium: 55 mg, Potassium: 400 mg, Cholesterol: 0 mg

Baked Beetroot Chips with Rosemary Salt

Preparation Time: 10 min.
Cooking Time: 25 min.
Mode of Cooking: Baking
Servings: 4
Ingredients:

- 3 large beetroots, thinly sliced
- 2 Tbsp olive oil
- 1 Tbsp chopped rosemary
- 1 tsp sea salt
- ½ tsp freshly ground pepper

Directions:

2. Preheat oven to 375°F (190°C)
3. Mix sliced beetroots with olive oil, chopped rosemary, sea salt, and pepper

- Arrange in a single layer on a baking tray
- Bake until crispy, about 20-25 min., turning halfway through

Tips:

- Use a mandoline slicer for evenly thin beetroot slices
- Pat beet slices dry with paper towels before seasoning to ensure crispiness

Nutritional Values: Calories: 110, Fat: 7g, Carbs: 10g, Protein: 2g, Sugar: 7g, Sodium: 600 mg, Potassium: 340 mg, Cholesterol: 0 mg

Garlic Thyme Stuffed Mushrooms

Preparation Time: 15 min.
Cooking Time: 20 min.
Mode of Cooking: Baking
Servings: 4
Ingredients:

- 12 large button mushrooms, stems removed
- 4 cloves garlic, minced

- 2 Tbsp olive oil
- 1 tsp dried thyme
- ¼ cup breadcrumbs
- ¼ cup grated Parmesan cheese
- Salt and pepper to taste

Directions:

1. Preheat oven to 375°F (190°C)
2. In a bowl, mix the minced garlic, olive oil, thyme, breadcrumbs, Parmesan, salt, and pepper
3. Stuff each mushroom cap with the breadcrumb mixture

- Arrange stuffed mushrooms on a baking dish
- Bake until the mushrooms are tender and the tops are golden brown, about 20 min.

Tips:

- For a gluten-free version, use almond meal instead of breadcrumbs
- Serve hot as an appetizer or side dish

Nutritional Values: Calories: 130, Fat: 9g, Carbs: 9g, Protein: 4g, Sugar: 2g, Sodium: 210 mg, Potassium: 300 mg, Cholesterol: 5 mg

Grilled Zucchini Ribbons with Lemon and Feta

Preparation Time: 15 min
Cooking Time: 10 min
Mode of Cooking: Grilling
Servings: 4
Ingredients:

- 3 medium zucchini, sliced into ribbons with a vegetable peeler
- 2 Tbsp olive oil
- 1 lemon, zested and juiced
- 1 clove garlic, minced
- Salt and freshly ground black pepper to taste
- ½ cup crumbled feta cheese
- 2 Tbsp fresh mint, chopped

Directions:

1. Preheat grill to medium-high (around 375°F (190°C))
2. In a bowl, toss zucchini ribbons with olive oil, garlic, lemon zest, and juice
3. Season with salt and pepper
4. Grill zucchini ribbons in a single layer, turning once, until tender and grill marks appear, about 2-3 min per side
5. Transfer to a serving platter, sprinkle with feta and mint

Tips:

- Serve immediately for best flavor and texture
- Add a drizzle of extra-virgin olive oil before serving for added richness

Nutritional Values: Calories: 150, Fat: 11g, Carbs: 9g, Protein: 7g, Sugar: 4g, Sodium: 320 mg, Potassium: 475 mg, Cholesterol: 25 mg

Quick Appetizers for Spontaneous Gatherings

Spicy Edamame-Guacamole Dip

Preparation Time: 10 min
Cooking Time: none
Mode of Cooking: No Cooking
Servings: 8
Ingredients:

- 1 C. edamame, shelled and cooked
- 2 ripe avocados, peeled and pitted
- 1 small red onion, finely chopped
- 1 jalapeño, seeded and minced
- 1 handful of fresh cilantro, chopped
- Juice of 1 lime
- 1 tsp salt
- 1/2 tsp black pepper

Directions:

1. Mash avocados and edamame together until they reach a coarse texture
2. Stir in red onion, jalapeño, cilantro, lime juice, salt, and black pepper until well mixed

Tips:

- Serve with sliced cucumbers or whole-grain crackers for a healthier option
- Add a splash of olive oil for an extra smoothness and healthy fats boost

Nutritional Values: Calories: 150, Fat: 12g, Carbs: 9g, Protein: 5g, Sugar: 2g, Sodium: 300 mg, Potassium: 450 mg, Cholesterol: 0 mg

Mini Portobello Pizzas

Preparation Time: 15 min
Cooking Time: 10 min
Mode of Cooking: Baking
Servings: 12
Ingredients:

- 12 mini Portobello mushrooms, stems removed
- 1 C. marinara sauce, no sugar added
- 1 C. shredded mozzarella cheese
- 1/2 C. cherry tomatoes, halved
- 1/4 C. black olives, sliced
- 2 Tbsp fresh basil, chopped
- Salt and pepper to taste

Directions:

1. Preheat oven to 375°F (190°C)
2. Arrange mushroom caps on a baking sheet
3. Spoon marinara sauce into each cap, then sprinkle with mozzarella, tomatoes, olives, and basil
4. Season with salt and pepper
5. Bake until cheese is bubbly, about 10 min

Tips:

- Use a variety of colored cherry tomatoes for a vibrant presentation
- Consider adding a sprinkle of nutritional yeast for an added cheesy flavor without extra dairy

Nutritional Values: Calories: 125, Fat: 9g, Carbs: 6g, Protein: 8g, Sugar: 3g, Sodium: 200 mg, Potassium: 360 mg, Cholesterol: 15 mg

Cucumber Roll-Ups with Hummus and Avocado

Preparation Time: 15 min
Cooking Time: none
Mode of Cooking: No Cooking
Servings: 10
Ingredients:

- 10 long cucumber strips, thinly sliced with a mandoline
- 1 C. hummus
- 1 avocado, thinly sliced
- 1 carrot, julienned
- 1 bell pepper, color of choice, julienned
- 1/4 C. alfalfa sprouts

Directions:

1. Lay cucumber strips flat on a clean surface
2. Spread a thin layer of hummus on each strip
3. Top with slices of avocado, julienned carrot, bell pepper, and sprouts
4. Carefully roll up the strips tightly

Tips:

- Chill the roll-ups in the refrigerator for 10 min before serving to firm them up
- Drizzle with lemon juice right before serving to add a fresh taste

Nutritional Values: Calories: 85, Fat: 5g, Carbs: 7g, Protein: 3g, Sugar: 1g, Sodium: 125 mg, Potassium: 270 mg, Cholesterol: 0 mg

Smoked Salmon and Dill Cream Cheese Canapes

Preparation Time: 20 min
Cooking Time: none
Mode of Cooking: No Cooking
Servings: 20
Ingredients:

- 1 French baguette, sliced into 20 pieces
- 4 oz smoked salmon, cut into small pieces
- 1/2 C. cream cheese, softened
- 2 Tbsp fresh dill, chopped
- 1 tsp lemon zest
- Black pepper to taste

Directions:

1. Mix cream cheese, dill, lemon zest, and black pepper in a bowl until well combined
2. Spread the dill cream cheese mixture on each baguette slice
3. Top with a piece of smoked salmon

Tips:

- Serve immediately or cover and chill until serving to allow flavors to meld
- Opt for wild-caught salmon for better flavor and health benefits

Nutritional Values: Calories: 110, Fat: 6g, Carbs: 9g, Protein: 7g, Sugar: 1g, Sodium: 180 mg, Potassium: 105 mg, Cholesterol: 20 mg

Chickpea and Sweet Potato Sliders

Preparation Time: 20 min
Cooking Time: 30 min
Mode of Cooking: Baking
Servings: 15
Ingredients:

- 2 C. sweet potatoes, peeled and grated
- 1 C. chickpeas, rinsed and mashed
- 1/4 C. red onion, finely chopped
- 2 cloves garlic, minced
- 1 tsp cumin
- 1 tsp paprika
- Salt and pepper to taste
- Olive oil for brushing

Directions:

1. Preheat oven to 375°F (190°C)
2. Combine all ingredients except olive oil in a large bowl
3. Shape mixture into small, flat patties
4. Place on a greased baking sheet
5. Brush each with olive oil
6. Bake until golden, about 30 min

Tips:

- Serve on mini whole-grain buns with a dollop of guacamole
- These sliders can be made in advance and reheated for quick serving

Nutritional Values: Calories: 140, Fat: 3g, Carbs: 22g, Protein: 5g, Sugar: 5g, Sodium: 200 mg, Potassium: 330 mg, Cholesterol: 0 mg

Chilled Cucumber Avocado Soup with Dill

Preparation Time: 15 min
Cooking Time: none
Mode of Cooking: Blending
Servings: 4
Ingredients:

- 2 large cucumbers, peeled and chopped
- 1 ripe avocado, pitted and scooped
- 1 garlic clove, minced
- 2 Tbsp fresh dill, chopped
- 1 cup plain yogurt, low-fat
- Juice of 1 lemon
- 1 tsp sea salt
- 1/4 tsp black pepper
- 1/2 cup cold water
- Dill sprigs for garnish

Directions:

1. Combine cucumbers, avocado, garlic, chopped dill, yogurt, lemon juice, sea salt, black pepper, and water in a blender
2. Blend until smooth
3. Chill in the refrigerator for at least 1 hr before serving
4. Serve garnished with dill sprigs

Tips:

- Serve with a side of whole-grain crackers for added texture and fiber
- Add a drizzle of extra virgin olive oil before serving to enhance the flavors and add healthy fats

Nutritional Values: Calories: 138, Fat: 9g, Carbs: 12g, Protein: 4g, Sugar: 6g, Sodium: 587 mg, Potassium: 517 mg, Cholesterol: 8 mg

11.Comfort in Every Spoon: Soup and Stew Recipes

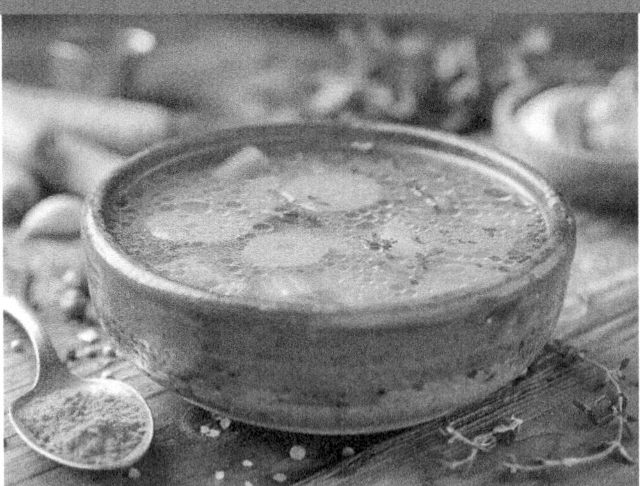

There's something inherently comforting about holding a warm bowl of soup or stew. It's like receiving a gentle hug from the inside, especially during a time when your body is undergoing significant changes such as menopause. Soups and stews can be both healing and heartening, offering deep nourishment while soothing common ailments that come with hormonal shifts.

In the realm of menopausal nutrition, the power of soup and stew goes beyond simple comfort. These dishes are excellent vehicles for delivering key nutrients that support hormonal balance and reduce inflammation. Imagine a broth teeming with anti-inflammatory ginger, turmeric, and garlic; these are not just ingredients but your allies in achieving wellness. With every spoonful, you're embraced by layers of flavor that also help manage the symptoms of menopause, such as hot flashes and mood swings. Preparing these recipes can be as therapeutic as consuming them. The process of chopping vegetables, simmering broths, and blending fresh herbs allows you to reconnect with the food you eat, understanding where it comes from and the benefits it brings. This connection deepens your relationship with your diet, turning each meal into an opportunity for self-care.

This chapter is not just about giving you recipes but about inviting you to embrace this tranquil ritual of cooking and enjoying soups and stews. From light, refreshing broths perfect for spring days to rich, creamy soups that shield you from winter's chill, each recipe is crafted to support your health at every stage of menopause.

Moreover, these dishes are wonderfully versatile and family-friendly. They can be easily adapted to suit different dietary needs and preferences, ensuring that everyone at your table can enjoy the same nutritious, comforting meal. This congruence between your needs and your family's enhances shared meal times, making them not just nutritious but also joyous occasions.

So, let us delve into the warm, inviting world of soups and stews together, spoon by spoon building towards a more balanced, healthy menopausal journey.

Health-Enhancing Broths

Golden Turmeric Bone Broth

Preparation Time: 10 min.

Cooking Time: 8 hr.

Mode of Cooking: Slow Cooking

Servings: 4

Ingredients:

- 2 lb. grass-fed beef bones
- 1 onion, quartered
- 4 cloves garlic, smashed
- 3 Tbsp apple cider vinegar
- 2 carrots, chopped
- 2 celery stalks, chopped
- 1 Tbsp turmeric powder
- 1 tsp freshly ground black pepper
- 1 gallon water
- 1 bay leaf

Directions:

1. Place beef bones in a slow cooker
2. Add onion, garlic, apple cider vinegar, carrots, celery, turmeric, black pepper, and bay leaf
3. Cover with water
4. Set to low and cook for 8 hr.
5. Strain the broth and discard solids

Tips:

- Store broth in jars in the fridge for quick use throughout the week

- Add a pinch of sea salt when serving to enhance flavor
- Can be frozen for up to 3 months

Nutritional Values: Calories: 40, Fat: 0g, Carbs: 3g, Protein: 6g, Sugar: 1g, Sodium: 58 mg, Potassium: 347 mg, Cholesterol: 0 mg

Healing Ginger Miso Broth

Preparation Time: 5 min.

Cooking Time: 25 min.

Mode of Cooking: Boiling

Servings: 6

Ingredients:

- 6 cups water
- 4 Tbsp miso paste
- 1 inch ginger root, thinly sliced
- 2 Tbsp tamari sauce
- 2 scallions, chopped
- 1 Tbsp sesame oil
- 1 tsp chili flakes
- ½ cup shiitake mushrooms, sliced

Directions:

1. Bring water to a boil
2. Reduce heat and add ginger and simmer for 10 min.
3. Remove ginger and dissolve miso paste in the broth
4. Add tamari, scallions, sesame oil, chili flakes, and shiitake mushrooms
5. Simmer for 15 min.

Tips:

- Serve hot and add a few drops of lemon juice for an extra tang
- Ideal as a base for vegetarian soup recipes
- Add tofu cubes for a protein boost

Nutritional Values: Calories: 70, Fat: 3g, Carbs: 7g, Protein: 3g, Sugar: 2g, Sodium: 940 mg, Potassium: 211 mg, Cholesterol: 0 mg

Soothing Lemongrass Coconut Broth

Preparation Time: 10 min.

Cooking Time: 30 min.

Mode of Cooking: Simmering

Servings: 4

Ingredients:

- 4 cups chicken broth
- 1 can (14 oz.) coconut milk
- 2 stalks lemongrass, smashed
- 3 kaffir lime leaves
- 1 Tbsp fish sauce
- 1 tsp sugar
- 1 small chili, sliced
- ½ cup cilantro, chopped
- 1 lime, juiced

Directions:

1. Combine chicken broth, coconut milk, lemongrass, kaffir lime leaves in a pot and bring to a simmer
2. Add fish sauce, sugar, and chili
3. Simmer for 20 min.
4. Remove from heat and stir in cilantro and lime juice

Tips:

- Can be used as a flavorful base for seafood soups
- Strain the broth before adding additional ingredients for a clearer soup
- Adjust chili amount according to spice preference

Nutritional Values: Calories: 150, Fat: 12g, Carbs: 8g, Protein: 3g, Sugar: 3g, Sodium: 400 mg, Potassium: 200 mg, Cholesterol: 0 mg

Nourishing Beetroot and Ginger Broth

Preparation Time: 15 min.

Cooking Time: 1 hr.

Mode of Cooking: Slow Simmer

Servings: 5

Ingredients:

- 3 medium beetroots, peeled and diced
- 1 Tbsp olive oil
- 1 onion, diced
- 3 cloves garlic, minced
- 2 tsp ginger, grated
- 5 cups vegetable stock
- 1 tsp salt
- ½ tsp black pepper
- 2 Tbsp lemon juice

Directions:

1. Heat olive oil in a pot and sauté onion, garlic, and ginger until soft
2. Add diced beetroots and cook for 5 min.
3. Pour in vegetable stock and season with salt and pepper
4. Simmer on low heat for 1 hr.
5. Stir in lemon juice before serving

Tips:

- Serve hot or cold depending on preference
- Excellent source of antioxidants
- Blend for a smoother texture if desired

Nutritional Values: Calories: 90, Fat: 4g, Carbs: 12g, Protein: 2g, Sugar: 7g, Sodium: 800 mg, Potassium: 370 mg, Cholesterol: 0 mg

Detoxing Parsley and Celery Broth

Preparation Time: 10 min.
Cooking Time: 40 min.
Mode of Cooking: Boiling
Servings: 4
Ingredients:

- 1 bunch parsley, chopped
- 4 celery stalks, chopped
- 1 lemon, halved
- 6 cups water
- 1 Tbsp apple cider vinegar
- 1 tsp sea salt
- ½ tsp cracked black pepper

Directions:

1. Combine all ingredients in a large pot and bring to a boil
2. Reduce heat and simmer for 40 min.
3. Strain the broth, squeezing the lemon halves into it before discarding

Tips:

- Refreshingly light
- Perfect as a detox or cleansing broth
- Add a pinch of cayenne pepper for an extra kick

Nutritional Values: Calories: 15, Fat: 0g, Carbs: 3g, Protein: 1g, Sugar: 1g, Sodium: 590 mg, Potassium: 300 mg, Cholesterol: 0 mg

Soothing Lemon and Thyme Chicken Broth

Preparation Time: 10 min
Cooking Time: 3 hr
Mode of Cooking: Slow Cooking
Servings: 6
Ingredients:

- 1 whole chicken, about 4 lb.
- 1 lemon, halved
- 4 sprigs fresh thyme
- 1 onion, halved
- 2 carrots, chopped
- 2 stalks celery, chopped
- 8 cups water
- Salt and pepper to taste

Directions:

1. Place chicken, lemon, thyme, onion, carrots, celery, and water in a large slow cooker
2. Cook on low for 3 hours
3. Remove chicken, strain broth, and season with salt and pepper

Tips:

- Add cooked, shredded chicken back into the broth for a heartier dish
- Broth can be used as a base for soups or sauces
- Store in the refrigerator for up to 5 days

Nutritional Values: Calories: 120, Fat: 3g, Carbs: 4g, Protein: 18g, Sugar: 2g, Sodium: 95 mg, Potassium: 250 mg, Cholesterol: 50 mg

Seasonal Creamy Soups

Autumn Butternut Squash Bisque

Preparation Time: 20 min.
Cooking Time: 40 min.
Mode of Cooking: Simmering
Servings: 6
Ingredients:

- 1 medium butternut squash, peeled and cubed
- 1 Tbsp olive oil
- 1 large onion, chopped
- 3 cups vegetable broth
- 1 cup light coconut milk
- 1 Tbsp fresh ginger, grated

- 1 Tbsp curry powder
- Salt to taste
- Freshly ground black pepper to taste

Directions:

1. Sauté onions in olive oil over medium heat until translucent
2. Add ginger and curry powder, stirring for about 1 min.
3. Introduce butternut squash and vegetable broth, bring to a boil and then simmer for 30 min. or until squash is tender
4. Blend the mixture until smooth using an immersion blender
5. Stir in coconut milk and season with salt and pepper
6. Heat through gently, ensuring not to boil

Tips:

- Serve with a swirl of coconut milk and a sprinkle of roasted pumpkin seeds for added texture and flavor
- Batch-cook and freeze in portions for a quick, healthy meal option

Nutritional Values: Calories: 175, Fat: 5g, Carbs: 30g, Protein: 3g, Sugar: 5g, Sodium: 505 mg, Potassium: 670 mg, Cholesterol: 0 mg

Creamy Cauliflower & Roasted Garlic Soup

Preparation Time: 15 min.

Cooking Time: 50 min.

Mode of Cooking: Roasting & Blending

Servings: 4

Ingredients:

- 1 head of cauliflower, cut into florets
- 1 bulb garlic, top sliced off
- 2 Tbsp olive oil
- 4 cups vegetable stock
- 1 onion, diced
- 1 tsp thyme, dried
- 1 cup almond milk
- Salt to taste
- Black pepper to taste

Directions:

1. Preheat oven to 400°F (200°C)
2. Roast cauliflower and garlic with a drizzle of olive oil for 30 min. until browned and tender
3. Sauté onion in remaining olive oil until soft
4. Squeeze roasted garlic out of its skin and add to pot along with cauliflower, onion, vegetable stock, and thyme
5. Simmer for 20 min.
6. Blend until creamy
7. Stir in almond milk, season with salt and pepper, and warm through

Tips:

- Use nutritional yeast for a cheesy flavor without dairy
- Roast extra garlic for future recipes or as a spread for bread

Nutritional Values: Calories: 160, Fat: 7g, Carbs: 22g, Protein: 5g, Sugar: 7g, Sodium: 480 mg, Potassium: 470 mg, Cholesterol: 0 mg

Winter Velvet Leek and Potato Soup

Preparation Time: 15 min.

Cooking Time: 35 min.

Mode of Cooking: Boiling

Servings: 5

Ingredients:

- 3 leeks, white and light green parts only, finely sliced
- 2 Tbsp butter
- 5 cups chicken broth
- 4 large potatoes, peeled and diced
- 1/4 cup heavy cream
- Salt and white pepper to taste
- Chives, chopped for garnish

Directions:

1. Melt butter in a large saucepan over medium heat
2. Add leeks and sauté until soft, about 10 min.
3. Add potatoes and chicken broth, bring to a boil, then simmer for 20 min. or until potatoes are very tender
4. Puree the soup with an immersion blender until smooth
5. Stir in cream, season with salt and white pepper
6. Serve hot, garnished with chives

Tips:

- Enhance flavor with a sprinkle of grated nutmeg
- Consider using sweet potatoes for a sweeter twist

Nutritional Values: Calories: 210, Fat: 8g, Carbs: 32g, Protein: 4g, Sugar: 3g, Sodium: 950 mg, Potassium: 721 mg, Cholesterol: 22 mg

Spiced Carrot Ginger Soup

Preparation Time: 15 min.
Cooking Time: 25 min.
Mode of Cooking: Simmering
Servings: 4
Ingredients:

- 2 Tbsp coconut oil
- 1 lb carrots, chopped
- 2 tsp ground ginger
- 1 onion, diced
- 4 cups vegetable broth
- 1 tsp cinnamon
- 1/2 tsp nutmeg
- 1 cup coconut milk
- Salt and pepper to taste

Directions:

1. Heat coconut oil in a pot over medium heat
2. Add onion and sauté until translucent
3. Stir in carrots, ginger, cinnamon, and nutmeg
4. Pour in vegetable broth and bring to a boil
5. Reduce heat and simmer until carrots are tender, about 20 min.
6. Blend the soup until smooth
7. Stir in coconut milk, season with salt and pepper, heat through without boiling

Tips:

- Serve with a dollop of yogurt and fresh cilantro for extra freshness and creaminess
- Garnish with toasted coconut flakes for a crunchy texture

Nutritional Values: Calories: 190, Fat: 14g, Carbs: 16g, Protein: 2g, Sugar: 6g, Sodium: 490 mg, Potassium: 430 mg, Cholesterol: 0 mg

Golden Butternut Squash and Ginger Soup

Preparation Time: 20 min.
Cooking Time: 45 min.
Mode of Cooking: Stovetop
Servings: 4
Ingredients:

- 1 medium butternut squash, peeled and cubed
- 2 Tbsp extra virgin olive oil
- 1 large onion, finely chopped
- 3 cloves garlic, minced
- 2-inch piece of ginger, peeled and grated
- 4 cups vegetable broth
- 1 tsp ground turmeric
- ½ tsp ground cinnamon
- Salt and pepper to taste
- Fresh cilantro and roasted pumpkin seeds for garnish

Directions:

1. Heat olive oil in a large pot over medium heat
2. Add onion, garlic, and ginger, sautéing until onion is translucent
3. Add butternut squash, turmeric, cinnamon, salt, and pepper, stirring to combine
4. Pour in vegetable broth, bring to a boil, then reduce heat and simmer for 30 min. or until squash is tender
5. Use an immersion blender to puree soup until smooth
6. Serve garnished with cilantro and roasted pumpkin seeds

Tips:

- Serve with a dollop of Greek yogurt for added creaminess
- Top with a sprinkle of chili flakes for a bit of heat

Nutritional Values: Calories: 175, Fat: 7g, Carbs: 27g, Protein: 3g, Sugar: 6g, Sodium: 500 mg, Potassium: 760 mg, Cholesterol: 0 mg

Creamy Parsnip and Apple Soup

Preparation Time: 15 min.
Cooking Time: 30 min.
Mode of Cooking: Stovetop
Servings: 6
Ingredients:

- 3 Tbsp unsalted butter
- 5 medium parsnips, peeled and chopped
- 2 apples, peeled and diced

- 1 large onion, chopped
- 4 cups chicken broth
- 1 cup light cream
- Salt and white pepper to taste
- Fresh thyme leaves for garnish

Directions:

1. Melt butter in a soup pot over medium heat
2. Add chopped onions, cooking until soft
3. Add parsnips and apples, cooking for 5 more min.
4. Pour in chicken broth and bring to a boil
5. Reduce heat to a simmer and cook until parsnips are soft, about 20 min.
6. Blend the soup until creamy using an immersion blender
7. Stir in cream and season with salt and white pepper
8. Serve hot, garnished with fresh thyme leaves

Tips:

- Add a pinch of nutmeg for a warm, nutty flavor
- Pair with a crusty whole-grain bread for a hearty meal

Nutritional Values: Calories: 220, Fat: 12g, Carbs: 28g, Protein: 4g, Sugar: 10g, Sodium: 300 mg, Potassium: 730 mg, Cholesterol: 35 mg

Refreshing Soups for Warm Weather

Chilled Cucumber Avocado Soup

Preparation Time: 15 min
Cooking Time: none
Mode of Cooking: Blending
Servings: 4
Ingredients:

- 2 large cucumbers, peeled, seeded, and chopped
- 1 ripe avocado, peeled and pitted
- 1 small shallot, peeled and chopped
- 2 cloves garlic
- 1 1/2 cups plain yogurt
- 2 Tbsp fresh lime juice
- 1/4 cup fresh dill
- 1/4 cup fresh parsley
- 1 tsp sea salt
- 1/2 tsp black pepper
- 1/4 tsp chili flakes
- 1/2 cup cold water

Directions:

1. Combine cucumbers, avocado, shallot, garlic, yogurt, lime juice, herbs, salt, pepper, chili flakes, and water in a blender
2. Blend until smooth
3. Chill in the refrigerator for at least 2 hrs before serving

Tips:

- Serve with a swirl of olive oil and a sprinkle of dill
- Can be stored in the refrigerator for up to 2 days

Nutritional Values: Calories: 184, Fat: 12g, Carbs: 16g, Protein: 6g, Sugar: 9g, Sodium: 597mg, Potassium: 550mg, Cholesterol: 7mg

Watermelon Gazpacho

Preparation Time: 20 min
Cooking Time: none
Mode of Cooking: Blending
Servings: 6
Ingredients:

- 4 cups cubed seedless watermelon
- 1 medium cucumber, peeled, seeded, and chopped
- 1 red bell pepper, chopped
- 1/4 cup chopped red onion
- 1 small jalapeño, seeded and minced
- 2 Tbsp red wine vinegar
- 1 Tbsp olive oil
- 1 Tbsp fresh lime juice
- 1/2 tsp sea salt
- Fresh herbs (mint or basil) for garnish

Directions:

1. Combine watermelon, cucumber, bell pepper, onion, jalapeño, vinegar, olive oil, lime juice, and salt in a blender
2. Pulse until finely chopped but not pureed

3. Chill for at least 3 hrs

Tips:

- Garnish with fresh herbs before serving
- Adjust seasoning with more salt and lime juice if needed after chilling

Nutritional Values: Calories: 70, Fat: 2.5g, Carbs: 12g, Protein: 1g, Sugar: 8g, Sodium: 200mg, Potassium: 169mg, Cholesterol: 0mg

Thai Coconut Cucumber Soup

Preparation Time: 10 min

Cooking Time: none

Mode of Cooking: Blending

Servings: 4

Ingredients:

- 1 large cucumber, peeled and chopped
- 1 14-oz. can light coconut milk
- 1 Tbsp Thai green curry paste
- 1 Tbsp lime juice
- 1 tsp ginger, grated
- 2 Tbsp cilantro, chopped
- 1 Tbsp soy sauce
- 1 tsp honey
- 1/4 cup water
- Salt to taste
- Sliced green onions and red chili for garnish

Directions:

1. Blend cucumber, coconut milk, curry paste, lime juice, ginger, cilantro, soy sauce, honey, and water until smooth
2. Season with salt
3. Chill in the refrigerator for 2 hrs
4. Serve chilled

Tips:

- Top each serving with green onions and chili slices
- Add a few drops of sesame oil for an extra layer of flavor if desired

Nutritional Values: Calories: 102, Fat: 7.4g, Carbs: 9g, Protein: 1g, Sugar: 6g, Sodium: 539mg, Potassium: 120mg, Cholesterol: 0mg

Peach Basil Soup

Preparation Time: 10 min

Cooking Time: none

Mode of Cooking: Blending

Servings: 5

Ingredients:

- 3 ripe peaches, peeled and diced
- 1/4 cup fresh basil leaves
- Juice of 1 lemon
- 2 cups unsweetened almond milk
- 1 Tbsp honey
- 1/2 tsp vanilla extract
- Pinch of salt

Directions:

1. Puree all ingredients in a blender until smooth
2. Chill thoroughly, at least 3 hr before serving

Tips:

- Serve with additional chopped basil
- Consider adding a dollop of Greek yogurt for added creaminess

Nutritional Values: Calories: 76, Fat: 1.3g, Carbs: 15g, Protein: 1.4g, Sugar: 12g, Sodium: 91mg, Potassium: 316mg, Cholesterol: 0mg

Cold Beet Orange Soup

Preparation Time: 15 min

Cooking Time: none

Mode of Cooking: Blending

Servings: 4

Ingredients:

- 3 medium beets, cooked and peeled
- 2 oranges, juiced
- 1 Tbsp lemon juice
- 1 Tbsp olive oil
- 1 tsp ground cumin
- Salt and pepper to taste
- 1/4 cup plain yogurt
- Fresh mint for garnish

Directions:

1. Blend beets, orange juice, lemon juice, olive oil, and cumin until smooth

- Season with salt and pepper
- Chill in the refrigerator for a minimum of 2 hrs
- Stir in yogurt just before serving

Tips:

- Garnish with fresh mint leaves
- Add a spoonful of sour cream or additional yogurt for a creamier texture if desired

Nutritional Values: Calories: 123, Fat: 3.7g, Carbs: 19g, Protein: 3g, Sugar: 14g, Sodium: 86mg, Potassium: 440mg, Cholesterol: 1mg

Chilled Cucumber and Dill Soup

Preparation Time: 15 min
Cooking Time: none
Mode of Cooking: No Cooking
Servings: 4
Ingredients:

- 2 large cucumbers, peeled and chopped
- 1 cup plain Greek yogurt
- 1 clove garlic, minced
- 2 Tbsp fresh dill, chopped
- 1 Tbsp olive oil
- 1 Tbsp lemon juice
- Salt and pepper to taste
- 1/2 cup cold water

Directions:

2. Combine cucumbers, Greek yogurt, garlic, dill, olive oil, lemon juice, salt, and pepper in a blender
3. Blend until smooth
4. Gradually add cold water to achieve desired consistency
5. Chill in the refrigerator for at least 1 hr before serving

Tips:

- Serve with a sprig of fresh dill for garnish
- For a vegan version, substitute Greek yogurt with coconut yogurt

Nutritional Values: Calories: 85, Fat: 4g, Carbs: 9g, Protein: 4g, Sugar: 5g, Sodium: 50 mg, Potassium: 276 mg, Cholesterol: 10 mg

12. Desserts: Sweet Conclusions

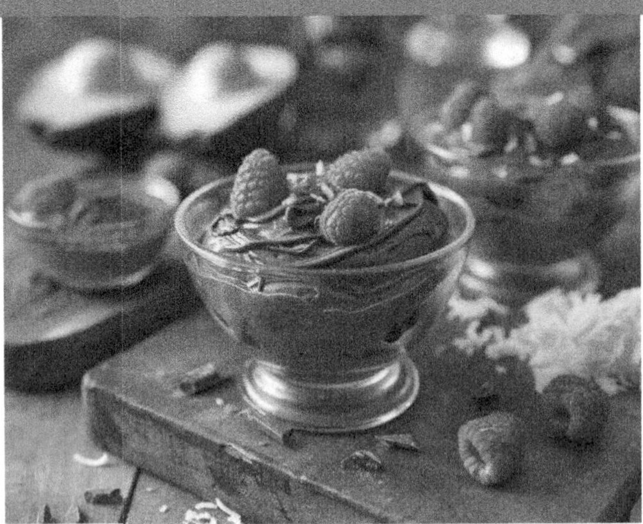

Imagine ending a delightful meal with a flourish of sweetness that doesn't spike your blood sugar or disrupt your well-managed diet. Yes, it is perfectly attainable, even during menopause, when it seems your body is in full rebellion mode. In this chapter, we turn the traditional notion of dessert on its head. Gone are the days when indulging in desserts spelled dietary doom, especially for those striving to balance hormones and control inflammation.

Navigating menopause doesn't have to mean foregoing the joy of a sweet ending to your meal. With a focus on anti-inflammatory ingredients and healthier alternatives, the desserts in this chapter are designed to cater not just to your taste buds, but to your body's changing needs. Each recipe here is more than just a treat; it's a celebration of balance and health, tweaked to enhance your menopausal diet rather than compromise it.

Consider the luxurious texture of a creamy avocado chocolate mousse or the refreshing zest from a berry and chia seed parfait. These aren't merely desserts; they symbolize an act of self-care, a way to honor your body's health while still engaging in the joy of eating. By incorporating ingredients like dark chocolate, rich in antioxidants, and substituting traditional sugars with natural sweeteners, these desserts help maintain hormonal balance without the typical guilt associated with sweet indulgences.

Moreover, the beauty of these recipes lies not just in their health benefits but in their simplicity. Many can be prepared ahead of time, making it easy to have a delectable treat at the ready without stress or significant time investment—vital for those busy evenings when yet another elaborate meal prep is out of the question.

So, as we explore these sweet conclusions, remember that each serves a purpose beyond mere pleasure. They are carefully crafted to ensure that your journey through menopause is not only healthy but also happy. Desserts can indeed be part of a balanced, health-forward lifestyle, providing comfort and celebration without detriment to your nutritional needs.

Healthier Baking Alternatives

Avocado Chocolate Mousse

Preparation Time: 15 min.
Cooking Time: none
Mode of Cooking: Blending
Servings: 6
Ingredients:

- 2 ripe avocados, peeled and pitted
- 1/4 C. raw cacao powder
- 1/4 C. high-quality maple syrup
- 1/2 tsp pure vanilla extract
- Pinch of sea salt
- 2 Tbsp unsweetened almond milk

Directions:

1. Combine avocados, cacao powder, maple syrup, vanilla, and salt in a blender or food processor
2. Blend until smooth, gradually adding almond milk to achieve desired consistency

Tips:

- Serve immediately or chill for an hour for thicker consistency
- Garnish with fresh raspberries or a sprinkle of shredded coconut for a touch of elegance and flavor

Nutritional Values: Calories: 184, Fat: 14g, Carbs: 17g, Protein: 2g, Sugar: 8g, Sodium: 8mg, Potassium: 487mg, Cholesterol: 0mg

Spiced Carrot and Quinoa Cake

Preparation Time: 20 min.
Cooking Time: 35 min.
Mode of Cooking: Baking
Servings: 8
Ingredients:

- 1½ C. whole wheat flour
- 1 tsp baking powder
- ½ tsp baking soda
- 1¼ tsp ground cinnamon
- ½ tsp ground nutmeg
- ¼ tsp ground ginger
- Pinch of salt
- ¾ C. cooked quinoa
- ¾ C. grated carrots
- ½ C. unsweetened applesauce
- ¼ C. olive oil
- 2 large eggs
- ¾ C. raw honey
- 2 tsp vanilla extract
- ½ C. walnuts, chopped

Directions:

1. Preheat oven to 350°F (175°C)
2. Grease and flour a 9-inch cake pan
3. In a large bowl, whisk together flour, baking powder, baking soda, cinnamon, nutmeg, ginger, and salt
4. In a separate bowl, mix quinoa, carrots, applesauce, olive oil, eggs, honey, and vanilla
5. Add wet ingredients to dry, mix until just combined
6. Fold in walnuts
7. Pour into prepared pan
8. Bake until a toothpick inserted into the center comes out clean, about 35 min.

Tips:

- Allow cake to cool in pan for 10 min. before turning out onto a wire rack to cool completely
- Top with a light dusting of powdered cinnamon for added flavor and presentation

Nutritional Values: Calories: 276, Fat: 11g, Carbs: 42g, Protein: 6g, Sugar: 22g, Sodium: 167mg, Potassium: 135mg, Cholesterol: 47mg

Almond Flour Lemon Bars

Preparation Time: 15 min.
Cooking Time: 25 min.
Mode of Cooking: Baking
Servings: 10
Ingredients:

- For the crust: 2 C. almond flour
- 1/3 C. coconut oil, melted
- 2 Tbsp maple syrup
- Pinch of salt; For the filling: 3 large eggs
- ½ C. honey
- ½ C. fresh lemon juice
- 2 Tbsp lemon zest
- ¼ C. almond flour
- Powdered erythritol, for dusting

Directions:

1. Preheat oven to 350°F (175°C)
2. Line an 8x8 inch baking pan with parchment paper
3. Mix almond flour, coconut oil, maple syrup, and salt for the crust until well combined
4. Press evenly into the bottom of prepared pan
5. Bake for 10 min.
6. Whisk together eggs, honey, lemon juice, zest, and almond flour for filling
7. Pour over baked crust
8. Bake until filling is set, about 15 min.
9. Cool completely
10. Dust with erythritol before serving

Tips:

- Store in the refrigerator for up to 5 days for best freshness
- Use organic lemons for a more vibrant flavor

Nutritional Values: Calories: 273, Fat: 20g, Carbs: 21g, Protein: 7g, Sugar: 15g, Sodium: 45mg, Potassium: 55mg, Cholesterol: 62mg

Pumpkin Seed and Oat Cookies

Preparation Time: 10 min.
Cooking Time: 12 min.
Mode of Cooking: Baking
Servings: 15

Ingredients:

- 1 C. rolled oats
- ¾ C. whole wheat flour
- 1 tsp baking powder
- ¼ tsp salt
- ½ C. pumpkin seeds
- ¼ C. sunflower seeds
- ¼ C. coconut oil, melted
- ½ C. honey
- 1 tsp vanilla extract

Directions:

1. Preheat oven to 375°F (190°C)
2. Line a baking sheet with parchment paper
3. In a bowl, mix oats, flour, baking powder, and salt
4. Stir in pumpkin seeds and sunflower seeds
5. In another bowl, whisk together coconut oil, honey, and vanilla
6. Combine wet and dry ingredients until just mixed
7. Drop spoonfuls of dough onto prepared sheet
8. Bake until edges are golden, about 12 min.

Tips:

- Let cookies cool on the sheet for 5 min. before transferring to a wire rack to cool completely
- These cookies can be stored in an airtight container to retain their crispness

Nutritional Values: Calories: 160, Fat: 9g, Carbs: 18g, Protein: 3g, Sugar: 9g, Sodium: 55mg, Potassium: 90mg, Cholesterol: 0mg

Baked Pear with Walnut and Honey

Preparation Time: 10 min.

Cooking Time: 25 min.

Mode of Cooking: Baking

Servings: 4

Ingredients:

- 2 large pears, halved and cored
- ¼ C. chopped walnuts
- 4 tsp honey
- ¼ tsp ground cinnamon
- 1/4 tsp ground cloves
- 1/4 cup crushed walnuts for topping

Directions:

1. Preheat oven to 350°F (175°C)
2. Arrange pear halves cut-side up on a baking dish
3. Mix chopped walnuts, honey, cinnamon, and cloves
4. Spoon mixture into the center of each pear half
5. Top with crushed walnuts
6. Bake until pears are tender, about 25 min.

Tips:

- Serve warm, perhaps with a dollop of Greek yogurt
- Pears can be baked a day ahead and reheated before serving

Nutritional Values: Calories: 150, Fat: 7g, Carbs: 22g, Protein: 2g, Sugar: 16g, Sodium: 2mg, Potassium: 170mg, Cholesterol: 0mg

Spiced Carrot Cake with Avocado Frosting

Preparation Time: 20 min.

Cooking Time: 30 min.

Mode of Cooking: Baking

Servings: 12

Ingredients:

- 2 cups whole wheat flour
- 1 tsp baking soda
- 2 tsp ground cinnamon
- 1/2 tsp ground nutmeg
- 1/4 tsp ground ginger
- 1/2 tsp salt
- 3/4 cup unsweetened applesauce
- 1/4 cup olive oil
- 3/4 cup maple syrup
- 2 large eggs
- 1 tsp vanilla extract
- 2 cups grated carrots
- 1/2 cup chopped walnuts

Directions:

1. Preheat oven to 350°F (175°C)
2. In a bowl, mix flour, baking soda, cinnamon, nutmeg, ginger, and salt
3. In another bowl, whisk applesauce, olive oil, maple syrup, eggs, and vanilla
4. Combine wet and dry ingredients
5. Fold in carrots and walnuts
6. Pour into greased baking pan

7. Bake for 30 min. or until toothpick comes out clean

Tips:

- Use ripe avocados for a creamier frosting
- Adding a pinch of salt to the frosting can enhance the flavors

Nutritional Values: Calories: 208, Fat: 9g, Carbs: 30g, Protein: 4g, Sugar: 11g, Sodium: 230mg, Potassium: 161mg, Cholesterol: 31mg

Homemade Frozen Desserts

Avocado Lime Sorbet

Preparation Time: 15 min
Cooking Time: none
Mode of Cooking: Freezing
Servings: 4
Ingredients:

- 2 ripe avocados, peeled and pitted
- Juice of 2 limes
- Zest of 1 lime
- 1/3 C. honey
- 1 C. water
- Pinch of sea salt

Directions:

1. Blend avocados, lime juice, lime zest, honey, water, and sea salt until smooth
2. Pour mixture into a shallow dish and freeze for about 2 hours or until nearly solid
3. Scrape the sorbet with a fork to create a fluffy texture right before serving

Tips:

- Serve immediately for best flavor and texture
- Adding a sprinkle of lime zest on top enhances flavor and presentation
- For a creamier texture, briefly re-blend the sorbet before serving

Nutritional Values: Calories: 210, Fat: 14g, Carbs: 22g, Protein: 2g, Sugar: 17g, Sodium: 20 mg, Potassium: 487 mg, Cholesterol: 0 mg

Coconut Matcha Ice Cream

Preparation Time: 20 min
Cooking Time: none
Mode of Cooking: Freezing
Servings: 6
Ingredients:

- 1 can (14 oz.) coconut milk, full fat
- 2 tsp matcha powder
- 1/3 C. honey
- 1 tsp vanilla extract
- Pinch salt

Directions:

1. Whisk together coconut milk, matcha powder, honey, vanilla extract, and salt in a bowl until well combined
2. Pour mixture into an ice cream maker and churn according to manufacturer's instructions
3. Transfer to an airtight container and freeze until firm

Tips:

- Store in the freezer in an airtight container
- Serve with a drizzle of honey or sprinkle of shredded coconut for extra flavor

Nutritional Values: Calories: 230, Fat: 18g, Carbs: 16g, Protein: 2g, Sugar: 14g, Sodium: 30 mg, Potassium: 80 mg, Cholesterol: 0 mg

Berry Basil Frozen Yogurt

Preparation Time: 10 min
Cooking Time: none
Mode of Cooking: Freezing
Servings: 4
Ingredients:

- 2 C. Greek yogurt, low fat
- 1 C. mixed berries (strawberries, blueberries, raspberries), fresh or frozen
- 1/4 C. honey
- 1/4 C. fresh basil leaves, finely chopped
- Juice of 1 lemon

Directions:

1. Combine Greek yogurt, mixed berries, honey, chopped basil, and lemon juice in a blender and blend until smooth
2. Pour mixture into an ice cream maker and churn according to manufacturer's instructions
3. Serve immediately or freeze in an airtight container to desired consistency

Tips:

- Garnish with additional basil leaves for a refreshing twist
- Pair with a sprig of mint for a nice color contrast and additional flavor
- Using frozen berries can help achieve a thicker consistency quicker

Nutritional Values: Calories: 160, Fat: 1g, Carbs: 28g, Protein: 10g, Sugar: 24g, Sodium: 45 mg, Potassium: 240 mg, Cholesterol: 5 mg

Pistachio Saffron Popsicles

Preparation Time: 25 min
Cooking Time: none
Mode of Cooking: Freezing
Servings: 6
Ingredients:

- 1/3 C. pistachios, unsalted and shelled
- 2 C. almond milk
- 1/3 C. honey
- Pinch of saffron threads
- 1 tsp rose water
- Pistachio slivers, for garnish

Directions:

1. Grind pistachios with a small amount of almond milk to form a smooth paste
2. Heat the rest of the almond milk in a saucepan with honey and saffron threads until honey is dissolved and milk is infused
3. Let cool, then mix in pistachio paste and rose water
4. Pour into popsicle molds, add pistachio slivers on the top, and freeze until solid

Tips:

- Dip molds briefly in warm water for easier removal of popsicles
- Infuse the saffron with warm milk for at least 10 minutes to enhance its flavor and color

Nutritional Values: Calories: 150, Fat: 8g, Carbs: 18g, Protein: 3g, Sugar: 17g, Sodium: 30 mg, Potassium: 115 mg, Cholesterol: 0 mg

Mango Chili Lime Sorbet

Preparation Time: 15 min
Cooking Time: none
Mode of Cooking: Freezing
Servings: 4
Ingredients:

- 2 large ripe mangoes, peeled and cubed
- Juice of 2 limes
- Zest of 1 lime
- 2 tsp chili powder
- 1/3 C. agave syrup
- 1/4 tsp salt

Directions:

1. Puree mangoes, lime juice, lime zest, chili powder, agave syrup, and salt in a blender until smooth
2. Pour mixture into an ice cream maker and churn according to manufacturer's instructions, then freeze until desired consistency is achieved

Tips:

- Add a pinch of extra chili powder before serving if more spice is desired
- The sorbet can also be made without an ice cream maker by freezing the mixture and stirring vigorously every 30 min until frozen

Nutritional Values: Calories: 200, Fat: 0.5g, Carbs: 50g, Protein: 2g, Sugar: 48g, Sodium: 150 mg, Potassium: 345 mg, Cholesterol: 0 mg

Mango Coconut Chia Freeze

Preparation Time: 15 min
Cooking Time: none
Mode of Cooking: Freezing
Servings: 6
Ingredients:

- 2 cups ripe mango, peeled and diced
- 1 can (13.5 oz) coconut milk
- 2 Tbsp chia seeds
- 1 Tbsp lime juice
- 1 Tbsp honey
- ¼ tsp vanilla extract

Directions:

1. Puree mango, coconut milk, lime juice, honey, and vanilla extract together until smooth
2. Stir in chia seeds thoroughly

3. Pour mixture into a shallow dish and freeze for 3-4 hrs, stirring occasionally until it reaches a sorbet-like consistency

Tips:

- Store in an airtight container in the freezer for up to one month for optimal freshness
- Serve with a sprinkle of lime zest for an extra zing
- For a creamier texture, blend again before serving

Nutritional Values: Calories: 200, Fat: 11g, Carbs: 25g, Protein: 2g, Sugar: 20g, Sodium: 15 mg, Potassium: 250 mg, Cholesterol: 0 mg

Quick and Healthy Sweet Treats

Matcha Coconut Truffles

Preparation Time: 20 min
Cooking Time: none
Mode of Cooking: No Cooking
Servings: 16
Ingredients:

- 1 C. unsweetened shredded coconut
- 1/4 C. coconut oil
- 1/4 C. honey
- 1 Tbsp matcha powder
- 1/2 tsp vanilla extract
- Pinch of salt

Directions:

1. Combine coconut, matcha powder, and salt in a bowl
2. Melt coconut oil with honey and vanilla over low heat, then pour over dry ingredients and mix until uniform
3. Refrigerate mixture for 10 min then form into small balls
4. Chill in refrigerator until firm

Tips:

- Use high-quality, ceremonial grade matcha for the best flavor and health benefits
- Can be stored in an airtight container in the refrigerator for up to a week
- Rolling truffles in extra shredded coconut or matcha can enhance flavor and presentation

Nutritional Values: Calories: 130, Fat: 11g, Carbs: 8g, Protein: 1g, Sugar: 6g, Sodium: 5 mg, Potassium: 30 mg, Cholesterol: 0 mg

Chia Raspberry Bites

Preparation Time: 15 min
Cooking Time: 1 hr chilling
Mode of Cooking: No Cooking
Servings: 20
Ingredients:

- 1 C. oats
- 1/2 C. chia seeds
- 1/4 C. almond butter
- 1/4 C. honey
- 1/2 C. fresh raspberries
- 1 tsp vanilla extract

Directions:

1. Mash raspberries smoothly in a bowl
2. Add oats, chia seeds, almond butter, honey, and vanilla extract and stir to combine well
3. Refrigerate mixture for 1 hr to set
4. Roll the mixture into bite-size balls

Tips:

- Store these bites in the refrigerator to maintain freshness
- Swap raspberries with blueberries or blackberries for a different flavor twist
- Pressing the mixture into molds can create fun, bite-sized shapes for special occasions

Nutritional Values: Calories: 95, Fat: 4.5g, Carbs: 12g, Protein: 3g, Sugar: 5g, Sodium: 15 mg, Potassium: 50 mg, Cholesterol: 0 mg

Pistachio Lemon Clusters

Preparation Time: 15 min
Cooking Time: 1 hr setting
Mode of Cooking: Freezing
Servings: 15
Ingredients:

- 1 C. shelled pistachios, unsalted
- 1/4 C. coconut flakes
- Zest of 1 lemon
- 2 Tbsp honey
- 1 Tbsp coconut oil

Directions:

1. Toast pistachios and coconut flakes in a dry pan until fragrant
2. Mix honey, coconut oil, and lemon zest in a saucepan over low heat until combined
3. Pour over pistachios and coconut, mix well
4. Spoon small clusters onto a parchment-lined tray and freeze until set

Tips:

- Use freshly grated lemon zest for the best flavor
- These clusters can be stored in the freezer in an airtight container for up to a month
- Drizzle with dark chocolate for added decadence

Nutritional Values: Calories: 100, Fat: 8g, Carbs: 6g, Protein: 2g, Sugar: 4g, Sodium: 0 mg, Potassium: 95 mg, Cholesterol: 0 mg

Spiced Pear Chips

Preparation Time: 10 min
Cooking Time: 2 hr
Mode of Cooking: Baking
Servings: 30
Ingredients:

- 3 ripe pears
- 1/2 tsp ground cinnamon
- 1/4 tsp nutmeg
- 1 Tbsp honey

Directions:

1. Thinly slice pears and arrange in a single layer on a baking sheet lined with parchment paper
2. Mix honey, cinnamon, and nutmeg in a small bowl and brush over pear slices
3. Bake in preheated oven at 225°F (107°C) until dried and crisp, about 2 hr, flipping halfway through

Tips:

- Choose pears that are firm but ripe for the best texture
- Sprinkle with a pinch of sea salt before baking to enhance the flavor
- Monitor closely as oven temperatures may vary, adjusting time as needed

Nutritional Values: Calories: 50, Fat: 0g, Carbs: 13g, Protein: 0g, Sugar: 10g, Sodium: 0 mg, Potassium: 75 mg, Cholesterol: 0 mg

Chia and Raspberry Pudding Cups

Preparation Time: 15 min
Cooking Time: none
Mode of Cooking: No Cooking
Servings: 4
Ingredients:

- 1/3 C. chia seeds
- 1 C. almond milk, unsweetened
- 1 C. Greek yogurt, unsweetened
- 1 Tbsp maple syrup, optional
- 1 tsp vanilla extract
- 1 C. fresh raspberries

Directions:

1. Combine chia seeds, almond milk, Greek yogurt, maple syrup, and vanilla extract in a bowl and mix well
2. Spoon half of the mixture into four serving cups
3. Top each with a layer of fresh raspberries
4. Divide remaining chia mixture among the cups
5. Refrigerate for at least 3 hrs to allow chia seeds to swell and thicken

Tips:

- Serve chilled topped with a few extra raspberries if desired
- Can substitute raspberries with blueberries or strawberries for variety

Nutritional Values: Calories: 180, Fat: 9g, Carbs: 20g, Protein: 8g, Sugar: 8g, Sodium: 30 mg, Potassium: 150 mg, Cholesterol: 10 mg

Golden Turmeric Energy Balls

Preparation Time: 15 min
Cooking Time: none
Mode of Cooking: No Cooking
Servings: 20
Ingredients:

- 1 C. rolled oats
- 1/2 C. shredded coconut, unsweetened
- 1/4 C. flaxseed meal
- 1/2 C. almond butter
- 1/4 C. honey

- 2 tsp turmeric powder
- 1 tsp ground cinnamon
- 1/4 tsp black pepper

Directions:

1. Combine rolled oats, shredded coconut, and flaxseed meal in a large bowl
2. In a separate bowl, mix almond butter, honey, turmeric powder, cinnamon, and black pepper until smooth
3. Add wet ingredients to dry ingredients and mix well
4. Roll the mixture into small balls

Tips:

- Store in an airtight container in the refrigerator
- Roll balls in extra coconut or cinnamon for additional flavoring

Nutritional Values: Calories: 100, Fat: 6g, Carbs: 10g, Protein: 3g, Sugar: 4g, Sodium: 10 mg, Potassium: 90 mg, Cholesterol: 0 mg

13. Implementing the Galveston Diet: 60-Day Meal Plan

As we turn the page to the practical implementation of the Galveston Diet, you now stand at a pivotal moment in your health journey. The next 60 days mark not just the transition into a meticulously crafted eating plan, but also a profound commitment to embracing a transformative way of life.

Imagine this phase as the bridge linking educated choices to tangible results. This is where theory meets practice and where you'll witness the positive changes that a well-structured diet plan can bring into your life. It's about more than just meals; it's about setting a new standard for health that resonates with the rhythm of your body's needs during menopause.

You might feel a mixture of excitement and nervousness as you ponder the changes ahead, which is perfectly natural. Remember those initial doubts and challenges shared among many women who have walked this path before you? They, too, faced the daunting task of altering lifelong eating habits and stepping out of their comfort zones. Yet, with each passing day, as they embraced the principles of hormone-balancing and anti-inflammatory foods, those small, consistent adjustments bloomed into rewarding lifestyle changes.

This chapter is designed to hand you the keys to the kingdom—an elaborate, day-by-day meal plan that respects your body's unique responses to menopause. Each week, you'll have a guide that anticipates your concerns, supports your body's fluctuating needs, and nourishes your soul. From energizing breakfasts to satiating dinners, every recipe has been chosen not just for its nutritional value but for its practicality and ability to integrate seamlessly into your daily routine.

As you embark on these 60 days, view each meal as an opportunity to fortify your body against the tides of hormonal changes. With every dish, you're not only feeding yourself but also learning to balance and recalibrate your body's needs. This journey is yours—unique in its challenges but also rich in potential for profound personal growth and well-being. Here's to stepping forward with confidence and curiosity, ready to transform not just your diet but your approach to menopause and overall health.

WEEK 1	breakfast	snack	lunch	snack	dinner
Monday	Golden Turmeric Smoothie Bowl	A handful of almonds	Mediterranean Crunch Salad	Sliced cucumber and hummus	Mediterranean Stuffed Salmon
Tuesday	Spinach and Feta Breakfast Scramble	Greek yogurt with a drizzle of honey	Roasted Beet and Citrus Salad	Carrot sticks with tzatziki sauce	Honey-Lime Baked Cod
Wednesday	Quinoa Apple Cinnamon Porridge	A small apple	Avocado and Quinoa Power Salad	A handful of mixed nuts	Lemon Garlic Shrimp with Zucchini Noodles
Thursday	Cocoa & Beet Detox Smoothie Bowl	Carrot sticks with hummus	Asian Sesame Edamame Salad	Celery sticks with almond butter	Balsamic Glazed Beetroot Wedges
Friday	Turkey and Quinoa Breakfast Bowl	A small bowl of mixed berries	Spicy Kale and Chickpea Toss	A few whole-grain crackers	Herb-Encrusted Chicken Parmesan
Saturday	Matcha Green Goddess Smoothie Bowl	A few slices of cheese	Roasted Beet and Arugula Salad with Walnuts	Fresh orange slices	Spicy Ground Turkey and Kale Stir-Fry
Sunday	Chia and Hemp Seed Yogurt Parfait	A handful of walnuts	Spicy Kale and Quinoa Black Bean Salad	A handful of baby carrots	Moroccan Lemon Chicken Tagine

WEEK 2	breakfast	snack	lunch	snack	dinner
Monday	Spirulina Protein Bowl	A handful of cashews	Herb-Infused Mushroom and Pea Pod Stir-Fry	Sliced bell pepper with guacamole	Citrus Herb Grilled Trout
Tuesday	Savory Spinach and Feta Breakfast Muffins	Celery sticks with hummus	Zesty Turmeric Roasted Cauliflower	A handful of pistachios	Spicy Grilled Tilapia with Avocado Salsa
Wednesday	Buckwheat and Chia Porridge	A small banana	Garlic Lemon Steamed Asparagus	Fresh orange slices	Baked Flounder with Lemon Butter Sauce
Thursday	Salmon and Avocado Omelette	A small bowl of mixed berries	Spicy Raw Carrot Ribbon Salad	A few whole-grain crackers	Mediterranean Herb-Grilled Salmon
Friday	Cottage Cheese Pancakes	Carrot sticks with almond butter	Charred Broccoli and Carrot Medley	A small apple	Citrus-Tarragon Baked Cod
Saturday	Acai Antioxidant Awakening Bowl	A handful of baby carrots	Steamed Ginger Scallion Bok Choy	Sliced cucumber with tzatziki sauce	Quick Garlic Butter Cod with Parsley
Sunday	Greek Yogurt Smoothie Bowl	A few slices of cheese	Balsamic Glazed Beetroot Wedges	A handful of mixed nuts	Spicy Shrimp Stir-Fry

WEEK 3	breakfast	snack	lunch	snack	dinner
Monday	Acai Antioxidant Smoothie Bowl	A handful of almonds	Mediterranean Crunch Salad	Sliced cucumber and hummus	Herb-Encrusted Chicken Parmesan
Tuesday	Chia and Hemp Seed Yogurt Parfait	Greek yogurt with a drizzle of honey	Roasted Beet and Citrus Salad	Carrot sticks with tzatziki sauce	Honey-Lime Baked Cod
Wednesday	Savory Turmeric Steel-Cut Oats	A small apple	Avocado and Quinoa Power Salad	A handful of mixed nuts	Lemon Garlic Shrimp with Zucchini Noodles
Thursday	Matcha Energy Bowl	Carrot sticks with hummus	Asian Sesame Edamame Salad	Celery sticks with almond butter	Balsamic Glazed Beetroot Wedges
Friday	Spiced Pumpkin Millet Porridge	A small bowl of mixed berries	Spicy Kale and Chickpea Toss	A few whole-grain crackers	Moroccan Lemon Chicken Tagine
Saturday	Savory Spinach and Feta Breakfast Muffins	A few slices of cheese	Roasted Beet and Arugula Salad with Walnuts	Fresh orange slices	Spicy Ground Turkey and Kale Stir-Fry
Sunday	Golden Turmeric Millet Porridge	A handful of walnuts	Spicy Kale and Quinoa Black Bean Salad	A handful of baby carrots	Mediterranean Stuffed Salmon

WEEK 4	breakfast	snack	lunch	snack	dinner
Monday	Matcha Green Goddess Smoothie Bowl	A handful of cashews	Herb-Infused Mushroom and Pea Pod Stir-Fry	Sliced bell pepper with guacamole	Citrus Herb Grilled Trout
Tuesday	Savory Buckwheat and Chia Porridge	Celery sticks with hummus	Zesty Turmeric Roasted Cauliflower	A handful of pistachios	Spicy Grilled Tilapia with Avocado Salsa
Wednesday	Cottage Cheese Pancakes	A small banana	Garlic Lemon Steamed Asparagus	Fresh orange slices	Baked Flounder with Lemon Butter Sauce
Thursday	Turkey and Quinoa Breakfast Bowl	A small bowl of mixed berries	Spicy Raw Carrot Ribbon Salad	A few whole-grain crackers	Mediterranean Herb-Grilled Salmon
Friday	Acai Antioxidant Awakening Bowl	Carrot sticks with almond butter	Charred Broccoli and Carrot Medley	A small apple	Citrus-Tarragon Baked Cod
Saturday	Spinach and Feta Breakfast Scramble	A handful of baby carrots	Steamed Ginger Scallion Bok Choy	Sliced cucumber with tzatziki sauce	Quick Garlic Butter Cod with Parsley
Sunday	Quinoa Apple Cinnamon Porridge	A few slices of cheese	Balsamic Glazed Beetroot Wedges	A handful of mixed nuts	Spicy Shrimp Stir-Fry

WEEK 5	breakfast	snack	lunch	snack	dinner
Monday	Golden Turmeric Smoothie Bowl	Greek yogurt with a drizzle of honey	Mediterranean Crunch Salad	Sliced cucumber and hummus	Mediterranean Stuffed Salmon
Tuesday	Spirulina Protein Bowl	A handful of almonds	Roasted Beet and Citrus Salad	Carrot sticks with tzatziki sauce	Honey-Lime Baked Cod
Wednesday	Acai Antioxidant Awakening Bowl	A small apple	Avocado and Quinoa Power Salad	A handful of mixed nuts	Lemon Garlic Shrimp with Zucchini Noodles
Thursday	Matcha Energy Bowl	Carrot sticks with hummus	Asian Sesame Edamame Salad	Celery sticks with almond butter	Balsamic Glazed Beetroot Wedges
Friday	Savory Spinach and Feta Breakfast Muffins	A small bowl of mixed berries	Spicy Kale and Chickpea Toss	A few whole-grain crackers	Herb-Encrusted Chicken Parmesan
Saturday	Chia and Hemp Seed Yogurt Parfait	A few slices of cheese	Roasted Beet and Arugula Salad with Walnuts	Fresh orange slices	Spicy Ground Turkey and Kale Stir-Fry
Sunday	Buckwheat and Chia Porridge	A handful of walnuts	Spicy Kale and Quinoa Black Bean Salad	A handful of baby carrots	Moroccan Lemon Chicken Tagine

WEEK 6	breakfast	snack	lunch	snack	dinner
Monday	Quinoa Apple Cinnamon Porridge	A handful of cashews	Herb-Infused Mushroom and Pea Pod Stir-Fry	Sliced bell pepper with guacamole	Citrus Herb Grilled Trout
Tuesday	Spinach and Feta Breakfast Scramble	Celery sticks with hummus	Zesty Turmeric Roasted Cauliflower	A handful of pistachios	Spicy Grilled Tilapia with Avocado Salsa
Wednesday	Matcha Green Goddess Smoothie Bowl	A small banana	Garlic Lemon Steamed Asparagus	Fresh orange slices	Baked Flounder with Lemon Butter Sauce
Thursday	Savory Turmeric Steel-Cut Oats	A small bowl of mixed berries	Spicy Raw Carrot Ribbon Salad	A few whole-grain crackers	Mediterranean Herb-Grilled Salmon
Friday	Turkey and Quinoa Breakfast Bowl	Carrot sticks with almond butter	Charred Broccoli and Carrot Medley	A small apple	Citrus-Tarragon Baked Cod
Saturday	Golden Turmeric Millet Porridge	A handful of baby carrots	Steamed Ginger Scallion Bok Choy	Sliced cucumber with tzatziki sauce	Quick Garlic Butter Cod with Parsley
Sunday	Greek Yogurt Smoothie Bowl	A few slices of cheese	Balsamic Glazed Beetroot Wedges	A handful of mixed nuts	Spicy Shrimp Stir-Fry

WEEK 7	breakfast	snack	lunch	snack	dinner
Monday	Acai Antioxidant Smoothie Bowl	A handful of almonds	Mediterranean Crunch Salad	Sliced cucumber and hummus	Herb-Encrusted Chicken Parmesan
Tuesday	Chia and Hemp Seed Yogurt Parfait	Greek yogurt with a drizzle of honey	Roasted Beet and Citrus Salad	Carrot sticks with tzatziki sauce	Honey-Lime Baked Cod
Wednesday	Savory Turmeric Steel-Cut Oats	A small apple	Avocado and Quinoa Power Salad	A handful of mixed nuts	Lemon Garlic Shrimp with Zucchini Noodles
Thursday	Matcha Energy Bowl	Carrot sticks with hummus	Asian Sesame Edamame Salad	Celery sticks with almond butter	Balsamic Glazed Beetroot Wedges
Friday	Spiced Pumpkin Millet Porridge	A small bowl of mixed berries	Spicy Kale and Chickpea Toss	A few whole-grain crackers	Moroccan Lemon Chicken Tagine
Saturday	Savory Spinach and Feta Breakfast Muffins	A few slices of cheese	Roasted Beet and Arugula Salad with Walnuts	Fresh orange slices	Spicy Ground Turkey and Kale Stir-Fry
Sunday	Golden Turmeric Millet Porridge	A handful of walnuts	Spicy Kale and Quinoa Black Bean Salad	A handful of baby carrots	Mediterranean Stuffed Salmon

WEEK 8	breakfast	snack	lunch	snack	dinner
Monday	Golden Turmeric Smoothie Bowl	Greek yogurt with a drizzle of honey	Mediterranean Crunch Salad	Sliced cucumber and hummus	Mediterranean Stuffed Salmon
Tuesday	Spirulina Protein Bowl	A handful of almonds	Roasted Beet and Citrus Salad	Carrot sticks with tzatziki sauce	Honey-Lime Baked Cod
Wednesday	Acai Antioxidant Awakening Bowl	A small apple	Avocado and Quinoa Power Salad	A handful of mixed nuts	Lemon Garlic Shrimp with Zucchini Noodles
Thursday	Matcha Energy Bowl	Carrot sticks with hummus	Asian Sesame Edamame Salad	Celery sticks with almond butter	Balsamic Glazed Beetroot Wedges
Friday	Savory Spinach and Feta Breakfast Muffins	A small bowl of mixed berries	Spicy Kale and Chickpea Toss	A few whole-grain crackers	Herb-Encrusted Chicken Parmesan
Saturday	Chia and Hemp Seed Yogurt Parfait	A few slices of cheese	Roasted Beet and Arugula Salad with Walnuts	Fresh orange slices	Spicy Ground Turkey and Kale Stir-Fry
Sunday	Buckwheat and Chia Porridge	A handful of walnuts	Spicy Kale and Quinoa Black Bean Salad	A handful of baby carrots	Moroccan Lemon Chicken Tagine

WEEK 9	breakfast	snack	lunch	snack	dinner
Monday	Quinoa Apple Cinnamon Porridge	A handful of cashews	Herb-Infused Mushroom and Pea Pod Stir-Fry	Sliced bell pepper with guacamole	Citrus Herb Grilled Trout
Tuesday	Spinach and Feta Breakfast Scramble	Celery sticks with hummus	Zesty Turmeric Roasted Cauliflower	A handful of pistachios	Spicy Grilled Tilapia with Avocado Salsa
Wednesday	Matcha Green Goddess Smoothie Bowl	A small banana	Garlic Lemon Steamed Asparagus	Fresh orange slices	Baked Flounder with Lemon Butter Sauce
Thursday	Savory Turmeric Steel-Cut Oats	A small bowl of mixed berries	Spicy Raw Carrot Ribbon Salad	A few whole-grain crackers	Mediterranean Herb-Grilled Salmon
Friday	Turkey and Quinoa Breakfast Bowl	Carrot sticks with almond butter	Charred Broccoli and Carrot Medley	A small apple	Citrus-Tarragon Baked Cod
Saturday	Golden Turmeric Millet Porridge	A handful of baby carrots	Steamed Ginger Scallion Bok Choy	Sliced cucumber with tzatziki sauce	Quick Garlic Butter Cod with Parsley
Sunday	Greek Yogurt Smoothie Bowl	A few slices of cheese	Balsamic Glazed Beetroot Wedges	A handful of mixed nuts	Spicy Shrimp Stir-Fry

14. Final Reflections: Embracing Your Health Journey

Reviewing Your Dietary Achievements

As we near the end of our journey together through the *Galveston Diet Cookbook for Beginners*, it's important to take a moment to reflect upon the strides you've made. This reflection is not just about patting ourselves on the back, although celebrating successes is certainly a part of it. It's more about understanding the depth and significance of our achievements, learning from our experiences, and fine-tuning our approach as we move forward.

Taking on a new diet, particularly one aimed at addressing the intricate dance of hormones during menopause, is no trivial task. You've embarked on this journey perhaps seeking weight management, alleviation of menopausal symptoms, or overall improved health. Whatever your initial motivations, by this point, you've spent several weeks recalibrating your body's responses to food, discovering new flavors, and probably challenging old culinary habits.

Understanding Your Achievements

Let us first acknowledge the shift in your metabolic understanding and its practical application in daily eating. You've learned how hormones play a central role in how your body functions and reacts to different foods, especially during menopause. The adjustments made in your macronutrient intake were designed not just to promote hormonal balance but also to reduce inflammation, which is often a silent aggravator of many menopausal symptoms.

These changes are subtle and often go unnoticed in the hustle of daily life. However, by now, you might have observed some signs that indicate enhancement in your metabolic health. Perhaps your energy levels have improved, or maybe those afternoon crashes are less frequent now. It's these little signals that suggest your body is responding well to your new dietary habits.

Navigating Challenges

Change, however, is rarely without its hurdles. Adjustments to your diet might have posed challenges, be it through dietary cravings, time management for meal prepping, or simply adapting to new tastes. Each challenge you faced was an opportunity—an opportunity to learn more about your resilience, to understand your body better, and to fine-tune your approach.

For instance, if you found yourself struggling with sticking to the intermittent fasting schedule, it provided an insight into your body's needs and perhaps pushed you to modify your fasting windows. These adaptations are crucial as they're not signs of failure but indications of your commitment to mold the diet to fit your unique lifestyle and needs.

Impact on Symptoms of Menopause

For many, the primary goal of adopting the Galveston Diet is to manage the uncomfortable symptoms of menopause. Reflect on this—how has your journey impacted these symptoms? Many women report reduced severity in hot flashes, more stable moods, and better sleep patterns. If you've noticed similar improvements, consider what elements of the diet may have contributed most significantly. Was it the reduced sugar intake, the increased fiber, or perhaps the more balanced eating schedules?

Family and Social Life Integration

Integrating a new diet into family and social life is often one of the biggest challenges but also one of the most rewarding achievements. Reflect on how your dietary changes have been accommodated during family meals or social gatherings. Your journey could have also inspired others in your household to make healthier food choices, a ripple effect that extends the benefits of your efforts.

Learning from Setbacks

It's also important to acknowledge and learn from any setbacks. Perhaps there were moments when you succumbed to old eating habits or skipped preparing meals due to a busy schedule. These are not defeats but are part of your learning curve. Each setback provides valuable insights into what works and what doesn't, helping you to build a more sustainable and enjoyable diet moving forward.

Sustainable Practices

Looking ahead, sustainability is key. Consider which practices and recipes you feel confident can be maintained long-term. Sustainability isn't just about persistence but also about enjoyment and ease. Which meals have become your favorites? What time of day do you enjoy eating the most on your new schedule? Recognizing these preferences helps solidify them into your routine.

Embracing Flexibility

Flexibility has hopefully become a cornerstone of your dietary approach throughout this journey. A rigid diet can lead to frustration and fatigue. Instead, learning to flow with life's unpredictabilities, adapting the principles of the Galveston Diet in a way that suits different days and different needs, can lead to lasting adherence and continued benefits.

What Lies Ahead

As you continue with this lifestyle, remember that diet is not just about controlling weight or symptoms but about nourishing your body in a way that enhances your overall vitality and well-being. The lessons learned, the habits formed, and the knowledge gained about nutritional strategies are tools that will stay with you, empowering you to make informed choices every day.

Reflecting on your journey, you've likely learned that dietary achievement is multifaceted. It encompasses physical health improvements, enhanced understanding of nutritional science, better coping strategies for managing symptoms, and a more harmonious integration of healthy eating into your social and family life. Each of these achievements is a stepping stone towards a healthier, more balanced you.

In conclusion, embrace these reflections as a testament to your hard work and as a guide shining light on how far you've come and where you can go from here. Your journey with the Galveston Diet is unique to you, filled with personal growth, health enhancements, and a deeper understanding of your body's needs during and beyond menopause.

Knowing When to Modify Your Diet Plan

Adapting our dietary choices to the ever-evolving tapestry of life requires an understanding that food is not just sustenance, but also a form of medicine that plays a crucial role in hormonal health, especially during menopause. The Galveston Diet, with its focus on hormonally balanced and anti-inflammatory foods, serves as a robust framework. However, the real art lies in knowing when and how to tweak this plan to continue meeting your body's changing needs. The journey through menopause is inherently dynamic. Symptoms and health needs can shift, sometimes subtly, other times significantly, as your body continues to recalibrate its hormonal environment. These shifts necessitate not only an initial adoption of new dietary habits but also periodic modifications to these habits.

Listening to Your Body

The first, and perhaps most important, indication that a dietary modification might be necessary comes from your body itself. Through this journey, you've likely developed a heightened awareness of how different foods impact your energy, your mood, your digestive functioning, and your menopausal symptoms.

For instance, if you initially found great success with a specific macronutrient ratio but now notice an increase in fatigue or resurgence of hot flashes, it might be time to revisit those ratios. It could also be the case that your sleep patterns have shifted, or your physical activity levels have changed, both of which significantly impact nutritional requirements.

Monitoring Health Markers

Apart from symptomatic cues, regular monitoring of health markers like blood sugar levels, cholesterol, and blood pressure can inform necessary diet modifications. Such clinical indicators provide a more objective measure of your body's response to your current diet. Should these markers begin to trend in unfavorable directions, it may be a signal that despite a diet's previous success, it needs adjustment to align with your current health status.

Experimental Adjustments

The idea of modifying your diet might seem daunting. A practical approach is to introduce small, experimental changes one at a time. Perhaps you might increase your intake of complex carbohydrates slightly to see if it impacts your energy levels, or introduce a broader variety of anti-inflammatory foods to see if this helps with joint stiffness experienced during menopause.

Documenting how your body reacts to these adjustments over a few weeks can provide insightful data that helps in making more permanent changes. This methodical approach reduces overwhelm and makes the process of adaptation less daunting.

Seasonal and Lifestyle Considerations

Your diet plan might also need modification based on seasonal changes or variations in your lifestyle. For instance, colder months might necessitate higher energy foods, or an increase in social activities might require more flexibility in your eating windows.

Furthermore, as you grow more active or possibly take on new physical hobbies, your body will demand different fuel types in different amounts. Acknowledging and adapting to these rhythmic changes in your life will not only improve your compliance with the diet but also enhance its effectiveness.

Emotional and Psychological Health

Diet affects more than just physical health—it's deeply entwined with emotional and psychological well-being. Times of high stress or emotional upheaval are not rare in menopause and can significantly affect dietary needs. During such times, a diet too rigid can add to stress, rather than alleviate it. Modifying your diet to include more mood-stabilizing foods, like those rich in omega-3 fatty acids, or allowing for small, pleasure-inducing treats can make the diet more supportive of your emotional health.

Aligning With Current Medical Guidance

Staying informed about the latest research in nutrition and menopausal health is crucial. What is considered a balanced diet today might evolve tomorrow based on new discoveries. Regular consultations with a healthcare provider, who can offer insights into the latest research, can guide necessary shifts in your dietary approach to ensure it remains optimal for your health.

Community and Support Adjustment

Finally, consider the role of social support in your dietary success. Changes in your social environment, such as a partner choosing to join you in your dietary plan, might require modifications to make the plan suitable for both of you. Alternatively, engaging with a community of women who are navigating similar health journeys can provide insights and inspire adjustments that you might not have considered.

Embracing the flexibility to modify your diet ensures that it remains a supportive, rather than restrictive, force in your life. Each woman's journey through menopause is unique, and so too should be her diet. By paying close attention to personal health signals, staying informed on medical advancements, and considering the broader context of lifestyle and seasonal changes, you can ensure that your diet continues supporting your health through menopause and beyond.

Developing a responsive approach to dietary planning is not merely about reacting to changes. It's about proactively crafting a lifestyle that continually fosters hormonal balance, reduces inflammation, and supports overall well-being. In doing so, your diet becomes a living, evolving entity that genuinely reflects and nurtures who you are in every stage of life.

Strategies for Maintaining Motivation

Embarking on a dietary journey, particularly during a transitional period like menopause, is akin to sailing: sometimes the waters are calm, and other times they are tumultuous. Keeping your sights set on the horizon—your health goals—requires maintaining motivation, even when the wind doesn't blow in your favor. Here are ways to cultivate and sustain this motivation over the long term, allowing you to reap the benefits of the Galveston Diet fully.

Connecting with Your 'Why'

The initiation of any new dietary habit often starts with a surge of initial enthusiasm. As time progresses, this excitement can wane. To counteract this, reconnect with your underlying motivations. Whether it's wanting to feel more energetic, manage weight, or reduce menopause symptoms such as hot flashes and mood swings, reminding yourself of these intentions can reignite your passion and commitment.

Consider writing down your reasons and placing them where you will see them daily. Each reason serves as a little beacon of light, guiding you back on track whenever your motivation dims.

Setting Realistic, Achievable Goals

Ambitious goals can be motivating, but they can also be daunting. Breaking larger goals into smaller, achievable objectives can help maintain momentum. For instance, if your goal is to incorporate more anti-inflammatory foods into your diet, start by introducing one new food a week. Small victories accumulate and each success strengthens your resolve to continue.

Celebrating Milestones

Throughout your health journey, it's essential to recognize and celebrate milestones. These need not be grand achievements; they could be as simple as sticking to your intermittent fasting schedule for a full week or mastering a new anti-inflammatory recipe. Celebrating these wins increases your sense of accomplishment, which fuels further commitment.

Simplifying Your Approach

Complicated diets often lead to frustration. Simplify your dietary approach by planning meals in advance and cooking in batches where possible. When your dietary regimen is straightforward, sticking to it becomes less burdensome, making it easier to stay motivated.

Visualizing Success

Visualization is a powerful tool for maintaining motivation. Regularly spend some quiet time envisioning yourself achieving your dietary goals. Imagine how you would feel and the things you would be doing differently. This mental rehearsal can boost your sense of self-efficacy and stimulate real-world implementation of your dietary intentions.

Leveraging Social Support

You do not have to walk this path alone. Sharing your goals with friends and family can create a support network that motivates you. Furthermore, consider joining online forums or local groups focused on menopause or nutrition. Such communities offer understanding, encouragement, and accountability, as members often share similar goals and challenges.

Seeking Professional Guidance

Sometimes, maintaining motivation might require the reinforcement of expert advice. Do not hesitate to consult with a dietitian or a healthcare provider specializing in menopausal health. These professionals can offer encouragement, adjust your dietary plan based on your changing needs, and help you navigate challenges effectively.

Embracing Flexibility

Rigidity can dampen your motivation. Life is full of surprises, and flexibility is critical. If you miss a meal or deviate from your diet plan, forgive yourself and get back on track with your next meal. Embracing flexibility rather than striving for perfection helps maintain a healthy relationship with food, reducing the risk of frustration and burnout.

Learning from Setbacks

Every journey has its setbacks. Instead of letting them deflate your motivation, view them as learning opportunities. Analyze what led to the setback and how it can be avoided in the future. This proactive stance not only aids in managing similar situations better but also fortifies your motivation.

Keeping the End in Mind

Finally, always keep the end in mind. Regularly remind yourself of the life-enhancing benefits of sticking with the Galveston Diet. Whether it's improved health metrics, better control of menopause symptoms, or simply feeling good in your body, keeping these end goals in sight can help sustain your motivation throughout your dietary adventure.

In essence, maintaining motivation on your dietary journey is about setting realistic goals, celebrating small victories, simplifying your approach, visualizing success, and leaning on social support. Equipping yourself with these strategies enables not just adherence to a dietary plan but the embracing of a lifestyle that continually champions your health and well-being. Each step forward, no matter how small, is a step towards a healthier, more vibrant you.

Lasting Advice for Sustained Health Success

As we draw curtains on our venture through the *Galveston Diet Cookbook for Beginners*, it becomes essential to glean lasting advice that transcends the specifics of any single diet or meal plan. Your journey towards managing menopause through diet does not end as you turn the last page of this book. Instead, it evolves into a more mindful approach to eating and living, which continues to nurture your body and mind long-term.

Embrace the Principles, Not Just the Plan

The real essence of sustained health success lies not in rigidly adhering to a prescribed set of rules, but in understanding and embracing the underlying principles. The core principles of the Galveston Diet—balancing hormones, reducing inflammation, and supporting overall health through nutrition—should be viewed as lifelong companions. These are not merely steps to be followed but wisdom to be lived by, adaptable to changing circumstances and stages of life.

Continuous Learning and Adaptation

The field of nutritional science is ever-evolving, and so are our bodies. Staying informed about the latest research and understanding how it applies to your personal health circumstances is crucial. Adaptation might mean adjusting your macronutrient ratios as your activity levels change, incorporating new anti-inflammatory foods into your diet, or tweaking meal timings to better suit your metabolic rhythm.

Intuitive Eating

Developing a sense of intuitive eating—listening to your body's hunger cues and eating accordingly—can profoundly shift your relationship with food. It breaks the cycle of eating according to the clock or a set plan and moves towards nourishment based on actual bodily needs. This practice encourages a deeper connection with your body and can promote more sustained health success by aligning your eating habits with your body's natural signals.

Holistic Approach to Health

While diet is a monumental aspect of managing health during menopause, it should be part of a broader, holistic approach to wellness. Include regular physical activity, be it yoga, swimming, or walking, into your routine. Don't underestimate the power of adequate sleep and managing stress through mindfulness or hobbies. A holistic approach ensures that you are not just feeding the body but also nourishing the mind and spirit.

Community and Connection

Sustaining health habits can sometimes feel isolating, especially if they seem at odds with the lifestyle of friends or family. Building a community, either online or in-person, with similar health goals can provide the necessary support and motivation to keep advancing on your health journey. Sharing experiences, challenges, and successes with others can not only enrich your own experience but can also provide encouragement and accountability.

Foster Flexibility and Kindness

It's vital to approach dietary changes with flexibility and kindness towards oneself. Strict regimens can lead to feelings of failure when deviations occur. Instead, foster a flexible approach where deviations from the diet are seen as part of the journey, not as setbacks. Permit yourself the kindness to enjoy an unplanned treat, then return to your usual eating patterns without guilt. This balance between discipline and flexibility can prevent feelings of deprivation and make your dietary changes more sustainable.

Reflect and Reassess

Regular reflection on what's working and what isn't can empower you to make informed adjustments that better suit your evolving needs. Perhaps you embarked on this journey with specific symptoms or goals in mind. As these change or as you achieve certain milestones, taking time to reassess and align your diet can help perpetuate your health successes.

Celebrate Your Journey

Finally, celebrate your journey. Each choice to eat a meal that supports your health, every bit of new knowledge about nutrition that you integrate into your life, and all moments of joy you find in this new way of eating contribute to a richer, more fulfilled you. Celebrating these achievements, both big and small, reinforces your commitment and fuels your motivation.

Long-term Success

Achieving sustained success in health through dietary adjustments is not an endpoint but a continuous journey of refinement and joy in eating well. You are not just following a diet; you are embodying a lifestyle, one which honors the dedication you have to your health and well-being.

Let the principles of the Galveston Diet illuminate your path, not just during the fleeting challenge of menopause, but as a lasting approach to living well. Embrace the journey with an open heart and a willing spirit, and watch as a new chapter of vibrant health unfolds before you.

SCAN THE QR CODE BELOW TO DOWNLOAD YOUR EXCLUSIVE BONUS:

7-DAY MENOPAUSE DETOX PLAN
HOT FLASHES TIPS AND SUGGESTIONS
40 PRINTABLE MINDFULNESS FLASHCARDS

Made in the USA
Monee, IL
02 September 2024